A Healthy Weight

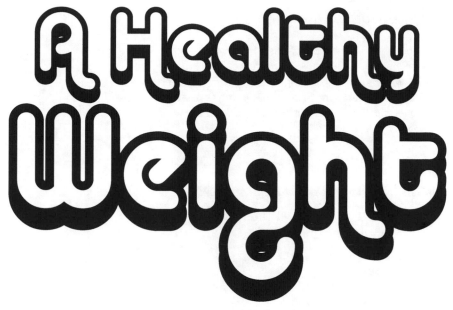

A Healthy Weight

The Best Birthday Gift
for Your Child

R. Matheny, PhD, RDN

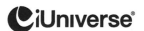

A HEALTHY WEIGHT
THE BEST BIRTHDAY GIFT FOR YOUR CHILD

iUniverse books may be ordered through booksellers or by contacting:

iUniverse
1663 Liberty Drive
Bloomington, IN 47403
www.iuniverse.com
1-800-Authors (1-800-288-4677)

ISBN: 978-1-5320-0699-9 (sc)
ISBN: 978-1-5320-0700-2 (e)

Library of Congress Control Number: 2016915975

Print information available on the last page.

iUniverse rev. date: 02/08/2017

In memory of and with love to my parents for their invaluable guidance and unconditional love throughout the years. Also in memory of Dr. Mary Frances Picciano, a wonderful scholar and researcher. Most of all, a thank-you to our Lord God and His Son for all that is meaningful in life.

Contents

Preface

One of my important dreams in life is to teach. My first attempt to do so took place in grade school during summer break. I invited some neighbor friends to come to my class. My loyal buddies came, but the love of having fun during the summer won over the spirit to learn. I thought my class was too short because it lasted only a few minutes. Life did continue.

Later, my years as a nutrition counselor in two health departments were rewarding. I enjoyed working with the families in the Special Supplemental Food Program for Women, Infants, and Children (WIC). Most of all, I believe that the medical checkups, coupons for nourishing foods, and nutrition advice helped expectant mothers have healthy babies and families raise healthy children.

In recent years, I have followed the reports of the Centers for Disease Control (cdc.gov/dataandstatistics). At present, millions of American adults, children, and teens are obese. With a large part of my education and professional experience in the area of public health, I wanted to help with the problem. I decided to use my teaching ability to write a book. The purpose of this book is to provide practical advice on how to prevent and correct obesity in infants, toddlers, children, and teens for mothers and fathers, caregivers, and expectant mothers.

I would like to share a memorable experience. At the health department, a preschooler wandered away from her mother, who was being interviewed by a clinic nurse. She quietly stepped into my room and began to chatter away. Two thoughts came to mind: "how precious" and "what a delight." My sincerest wish is that parents and caregivers put into practice this book's recommendations so that children, like this little girl, will have happy and healthy futures.

Acknowledgments

Warm thanks to my sister, Mary, and my brother, Bill, and his family for their continued support. My sincerest gratitude to Dr. Elizabeth Jones for her expert contributions, Sue Carson for her artwork, and my project coordinator and the editorial staff of iUniverse for their valuable recommendations to this book. Also, to Dr. Leann Birch for her class on child development and her assistance, along with Dr. Mary Frances Picciano for assistance with my PhD thesis in the area of breast-feeding and formula feeding. With great appreciation to Debra Scurry and Brenda Eads for their advice and technical assistance with the writing of this guide and to Ruth Flygare for proofreading the text. Also warm thanks to the staff of my local library, Robert Pierson and his assistants, Mary Becker, and Michelle Marvin for helping me acquire the professional resources required for the writing of this guide.

Introduction: Preventing Obesity as a Family Priority

The Role of Body Mass Index

In news reports on health, you often hear the term *body mass index*. What exactly is this index? Body mass index (BMI) uses an individual's height and weight to determine the total amount of fat in his or her body. The terms *overweight* and *obese* appear throughout this book. Based upon the Centers for Disease Control's standard growth charts (chapter 7), pediatricians consider a child to be:[1]

- *overweight* when his or her BMI value is in the range of the "85th to the 94th BMI percentiles for age" or
- *obese* when his or her BMI value is "at or above the 95th percentile for age".

The extra weight is responsible for the early appearance of serious medical and psychological problems among overweight and obese children and teens.

Becoming a Healthier Family

Regarding genetics, children are 40 percent more likely to be overweight or obese when one parent has a similar weight problem and 70 percent more likely when both parents do.[2] Although genetics contribute to the obesity problem, they *cannot* account for the dramatic rise in childhood obesity over the past several decades. Our modern environment exerts a stronger influence in terms of producing the weight problems among our nation's children and teens.

Children's eating and activity practices mirror those of their parents. Examples of today's unhealthy eating practices include the excess intake of foods high in fat, sugar, or salt; sweetened beverages; and large portion sizes of both foods and beverages. Similarly, examples of unhealthy activity practices include too much time spent with televisions and computers and the overuse of cell phones.

Because of these reasons, obesity is becoming a family concern, and weight management should be viewed as a family priority.

The significant role played by parents in establishing healthy practices in their children is emphasized throughout this book. You, as a parent, need to become proactive concerning matters of health.

The Purpose of the Book

The purpose of the practical advice in this book is to prevent or correct obesity in infants, toddlers, children, and teens. This advice will help you and your family acquire the five Hs: healthy weights, healthy minds, healthy dietary intakes, healthy eating practices, and healthy physical activity levels. The information in the chapters includes

- recommended feeding practices for infants;
- recommended dietary intakes for infants, toddlers, children, and teens;
- healthy eating practices for children and teens and for the family;
- healthy physical activity practices;
- normal growth, evaluating growth, and promoting a healthy weight in infants, toddlers, children, and teens;
- helping your family become psychologically fit; and
- setting healthy goals for the family and encouraging participation of children and teens in the family's meal-related activities.

This book will be helpful to expectant mothers who acquire such knowledge before the baby arrives, especially the chapters focusing on infants. The practical advice given in this book has been based upon the author's professional experience in the areas of infant and childhood nutrition and supported by the following reliable sources:

- nutrition expert, Dr. Elizabeth Jones, DED, MPH, RDN, FAND, and the American Academy of Pediatrics
- governmental sources, including the United States Department of Agriculture and the Centers for Disease Control
- websites that present educational information in a way that appeals to and holds the attention of children
- websites and other sources that provide related information that is not included in this book

Start by reinforcing healthy practices while correcting unhealthy ones. Good luck to you and your family on your journey to better health and a *fun* and *satisfying* way of life.

Endnotes

1   S. E. Barlow and W. H. Dietz, "Obesity evaluation and treatment: Expert committee recommendations," Pediatrics 102 (2007): S164–S192.
2   G. Schirmer, Preventing Childhood Obesity (Bedford, TX: Med2000, Inc, 2005)

Chapter 1

Recommended Infant Feeding Practices

Infancy is a dynamic time of life. Your baby will be busy. He or she will be experiencing a rapid rate of growth during the first year; discovering new flavors and textures in the foods and beverages offered; and acquiring the developmental skills to hold and drink from a cup, eat using a spoon, and enjoy finger foods.

The practical pointers on breast-feeding and formula feeding and healthy eating practices in this chapter will ensure that these three important milestones will be healthy ones for your baby during this special time of life.

Getting Started

Breast milk and iron-fortified formula are recommended for infants in the first year of life.[1] Iron-fortified formula is also recommended for mothers who are breast-feeding and supplementing with formula. It is best to continue nursing for at least three months in order to acquire a wide range of health benefits, such as

1. a natural balance in nutrients,
2. antibodies to protect against infections,
3. biological substances to mature the intestinal tract, and
4. close bonding between mother and her baby.

It is best to breast-feed infants "on demand." That is, feeding should begin when the actions of the infant suggest hunger and discontinued when the actions suggest that the infant is full (see chapter 2). In the beginning, however, if the infant is not always doing so, a breast-feeding mother may wish to encourage her infant to nurse at least on average every two hours until breast-feeding is well established. This practice helps prevent engorgement and mastitis (infection) of the breast.

While I was a university student, the Cooperative Extension Service asked me to write an educational pamphlet on breast-feeding for the families it served. While writing this pamphlet, I learned that there are two important feeding practices to keep in mind when you first start to nurse: (1) Be sure that your baby takes all or most of the colored area surrounding the nipple. This releases the milk and starts it flowing from the breast ducts in this area. (2) Alternate the breast with which you start nursing. This ensures that both breasts have enough milk for the next feeding. A common practice is to attach a safety pin on the bra strap above the breast at which to start the next feeding.

Many hospitals now provide a woman experienced in breast-feeding who will offer practical pointers (like the above and many others) to newly nursing mothers so that they can have a successful experience.

In the beginning with formula-fed infants, you may wish to start with two ounces of formula, increasing the amount if the infant desires.

As Your Infant Grows

The amount per feeding and the total amount of formula daily will increase. For both feeding methods, the amount of time between feedings will lengthen. During growth spurts, however, formula-fed infants will increase the amount of formula consumed, and breast-fed infants will increase the frequency of nursing. Over time, most mothers and infants settle into a regular pattern of feeding.

Another feeding practice to note is the length of feeding. On average, the length of feeding takes between fifteen and twenty minutes, both for breast- and formula feeding.

If your infant eats at a fast pace, reduce the amount of formula consumed (and therefore the risk of overfeeding) by purchasing bottles with nipples that have smaller openings. Alternately, mothers and fathers as well as caregivers may wish to even out the pace of feeding by removing the bottle from baby's mouth and pausing for several minutes over the course of feeding.

Though not ideal, breast-feeding mothers may wish to pause longer when the infant is transferred from breast to breast.

This *pace of eating* reminds me of my experience when counseling breast-feeding mothers at the health department. Someone came up with the idea to name infants based on the way they nursed. One group included infants who attacked nursing with great vigor; in other words, a fast pace of nursing. These infants were affectionately known as the little "barracudas."

Unhealthy Feeding Practices to Avoid

Based on my experience and that of noted nutrition expert Dr. Elizabeth Jones, I would like to bring to your attention a number of unhealthy feeding practices[2] that can cause overfeeding and dental decay.

Do not prop up the infant's bottle (containing formula, breast milk, juices, etc.) at any time. Propping the bottle can cause ear infections.

Do not enlarge the bottle's nipple in order to feed a mixture of formula and cereal (or other foods). This practice is often done to help the infant sleep through the night, but there is no evidence that this works. If you truly believe the cereal helps the infant sleep, offer a small amount of cereal by spoon along with the evening's formula feeding. Afterward, clean any teeth present.

Do not cover the bottle's nipple with sugar, honey, corn syrup, or sweeteners. This also applies to the practice of adding such sweetened items to infant cereals or water. Honey should not be given to infants before one year of age because honey can be contaminated with the bacteria that cause botulism.

Do not force a formula-fed infant to finish any remaining formula in the bottle.

Do not prompt infants to finish any uneaten baby/table foods.

Healthy Feeding Practices

Do wait to introduce infant foods until after four months of age. Pediatricians differ in terms of when foods are to be introduced, but earlier introduction has an increased risk for overfeeding and allergic reactions to certain foods, as well as developmental reasons.

The sequence and rate by which foods are introduced also varies among pediatricians.

Do introduce only one food with a single ingredient at a time. Add one new food every four to five days. This practice enables the parent or caregiver to determine a possible allergic reaction (such as rash) or intolerance (digestive problems) to new food. Multi-ingredient foods can be offered later, when each ingredient has been observed separately for such reactions.

Do realize that infants have an "innate preference for sweet and salty tastes."[3] There is no evidence for introducing vegetables first and then fruits. However, I would recommend when giving a fruit and vegetable *in the same feeding*, offer a vegetable first and then a fruit. In this way, the infant may develop this preference, which can continue into childhood. Be sure to include a variety of both vegetables and fruits.

Do realize that infants are often reluctant to accept new textures. To reduce the risk of rejection, *gradually expose* the infant to different textures. Begin with commercial baby foods or homemade pureed foods. Next, add commercial toddler and/or mashed or ground table foods. Then, introduce finger food and small, bite-sized soft pieces of food.

Do offer a variety of foods with different colors, tastes, shapes, and textures to infants and toddlers because "children like and eat what is familiar to them."[3] Infants and children are "predisposed to be neophobic and reject new foods."[3] Encourage the child to take a bite or two. If a food is rejected, try it again later. Offer a new food repeatedly; it may take many attempts for your child to accept it.

Do pay close attention to your baby when introducing new foods; some foods can cause choking. To help minimize choking risk, be sure the infant is sitting upright; a pillow or two may be needed. Sit facing the infant so that choking can be readily recognized. Foods that are most likely to promote choking include nuts, potato chips, fruits with seeds, popcorn, celery, raw carrots, fish with bones, tough meats, and small or hard candies.[2] Hot dogs also are known to cause choking.

Preparing Homemade Infant Foods

Dr. Elizabeth Jones and I would like to share some practical pointers on how to prepare homemade infant foods, if you wish to do so:[2]

- Be sure to clean all equipment and utensils, as well as surface areas upon which the food is prepared. Wash off fresh fruits and vegetables.
- Fresh or frozen vegetables are preferred, but if you use canned, drain off liquid and lightly rinse the vegetables.
- Fresh or frozen fruits also are preferred. Check the labels of frozen products for sugar content. If you use canned, select fruits that are *not* packed in heavy syrup.
- If table foods are used, remove the infant's portion before adding salt or sugar.
- Remove any skins, seeds, and fibrous material before preparing.
- Puree with a blender or food processor or mash well, depending upon the infant's age at which he or she can eat the food without choking.
- Distribute the prepared food into ice cube trays.
- Once frozen, release food cubes into a Ziploc bag; then date and label. A cube or two of the food can be a single serving, depending upon the infant's age.
- Use refrigerated infant food within forty-eight hours and frozen food within three months.

Endnotes

1 R. E. Kleinman, *Pediatric Nutrition Handbook* (Elk Grove, IL: American Academy of Pediatrics, 2009).
2 E. G. Jones, *Good Nutrition for Your Baby* (San Diego: the Foundation for the Children of the Californians, 2005).
3 L. L. Birch and J. O. Fisher, "Development of eating behaviors among children and adolescents," *Pediatrics* 101 (1998): 539–549.

Chapter 2

Recommended Dietary Intakes for Infants and Toddlers

The Centers for Disease Control (CDC) reported in 2011–2012 that 17 percent of US children and teens—12.7 million—are obese.[1] Thanks to the persistent efforts of First Lady Michelle Obama, there has been a decline in the percentage of obese preschool children, from 14 percent in 2003–2004 to 8.4 percent in 2011–2012.

It is time that we put the brakes on and prevent any further increase in childhood obesity. How? As a mother, father, or caregiver, you can establish healthy dietary practices during the early years, even as early as the introduction of infant and table foods. Also important is reducing the risk of overfeeding your infant by (1) paying attention to the types of foods, beverages, and portion sizes offered to your infant and (2) learning the actions of infants and toddlers that express hunger and being full.

These two feeding practices control calories and ultimately the weight of your infant or toddler. Also important is to correct a weight problem once it occurs.

In subsequent chapters, I will provide recommendations for establishing healthy dietary intakes and eating practices for children and teens, as well as how to increase physical activity while reducing the amount of time being inactive.

Importance of Standard Measurement Sizes

Learning standard measurement sizes can enable you to better recognize appropriate portion sizes for your children. In the beginning, you may wish to measure the serving sizes of your foods and beverages. Alternatively, you could separate a standard nest of measuring cups and set of measuring spoons and display them in a place near the table where you can easily visualize them. This will aid you in learning how to eventually identify correct portion sizes.

The following points may be helpful:

1. Purchase a standard eight-ounce measuring cup or a standard set of measuring cups. Notice the markings on the standard measuring cups—one-fourth, one-half, three-fourths, and one cup.
2. Glassware comes in different sizes. To measure how much fluid your favorite glass or mug holds, fill a standard eight-ounce measuring cup. For example, your mug may hold 1 1/4 cups, or ten ounces of fluid. (Don't fill glassware to the top; you need to allow for spillage.)
3. You may use regular flatware teaspoons and tablespoons, but avoid using the larger serving spoons. If you wish to be more accurate, you can purchase a standard set of measuring spoons.

Table of Equal Measurements

	3 teaspoons	1 tablespoon
1/4 cup	2 ounces	4 tablespoons
1/2 cup	4 ounces	8 tablespoons
3/4 cup	6 ounces	12 tablespoons
1 cup	8 ounces	16 tablespoons

Actions of Infants Who Express Hunger and Being Full

For both breast-feeding and formula feeding, it is very important that mothers, fathers, and caregivers learn the appetite-related actions of hunger and being full as shown by infants. The natural way of keeping calories under control is by preventing overfeeding.

The most common actions of being hungry include the following:

- crying
- opening his or her mouth to the breast, bottle, cup, or spoon
- turning his or her head toward the breast, bottle, cup, or spoon

With time, you will learn to recognize the difference between crying out of hunger and crying from other infant discomforts.

The most common actions of being full include the following:

- resting peacefully, closing his or her mouth to the breast, bottle, cup, or spoon
- turning his or her head away from the breast, bottle, cup, or spoon

Healthy Food and Beverage Intakes for Infants

Gradually increase the amount of foods in each food group until you meet the recommended amount for a one-year-old given here.[2]

Milk Group

Breast milk and iron-fortified formula are recommended. Formula-fed infants have intakes of 16 ounces during the early weeks that will gradually increase to 24 to 32 ounces at six months and then decrease to 24 ounces at one year of age.

Remember the following important points regarding the use of formula:[2]

1. Do not reuse formula that remains in the bottle.
2. Cover the formula can when refrigerated.
3. Use refrigerated formula within forty-eight hours.

Bread and Cereal Group

Four servings are recommended daily. Select from the following:

- 4 tablespoons of dry infant cereal
- 2–4 tablespoons mashed pasta, noodles, macaroni, or rice

- 1/2 slice toast or tortilla
- teething foods, such as 1–3 low-sodium saltine crackers (small crackers) or 1–2 graham cracker squares (large crackers)

Introduce the bread and cereal group with the following steps:

1. Start with single-grain (rice, oat, or barley) iron-fortified cereals.
2. Introduce wheat, mixed cereals, high-protein cereals, or Cream of Wheat at eight months of age.
3. Do not offer mixed cereals until each ingredient has been tested for an allergic reaction.
4. Start with a thin mixture (1 teaspoon of cereal with 1–2 tablespoons of breast milk or formula), and gradually thicken to an oatmeal-type consistency containing 4 tablespoons.
5. *Supervise* your infant when giving teething foods to prevent choking.

Fruit and Vegetable Group
Five servings are recommended daily. Select from the following:

- 4 ounces of juice
- 2–4 tablespoons of fruit
- 2–4 tablespoons of vegetables

Introduce the fruit and vegetable group with the following steps:

1. Begin with 2 ounces of diluted juice, such as apple (1 ounce juice with 1 ounce of water), and gradually increase to 1 or 2 ounces and then to 4 ounces of juice.
2. Don't offer citrus juices (such as orange) until after baby's first birthday because of the potential for allergic reaction.
3. If you give adult juices to your baby, select fresh, canned, or frozen. Try apple (1 ounce juice to 1 ounce water) or grape juice (1 ounce juice to 3 ounces water).
4. Offer *no more* than 4 ounces of juice daily. Water is the best choice as an additional fluid.

5. Offer juice in a spill-proof infant feeding cup, not in a bottle. When feeding commercial baby food, pureed home-prepared food, or table food, start with 1 teaspoon and gradually increase to 2–4 tablespoons of the fruit and vegetable.

Meat and Meat Alternatives
Four servings are recommended daily. Select from the following:

- 2–4 tablespoons of soft, cooked meat (lamb, poultry, or beef) or fish (no shellfish)
- 2–4 tablespoons of plain yogurt or cottage cheese
- 2–4 tablespoons of soft-cooked dried beans or peas (without skins)
- 1 slice of cheese
- 1 cooked egg yolk

Introduce the meat and meat alternatives group with the following steps:

1. Start with 1 teaspoon and gradually increase to 2 to 4 tablespoons.
2. Mix the cooked egg yolk with a little breast milk or formula; gradually decrease the liquid with each feeding until there is just the egg yolk itself. (Do not offer egg white or the whole egg until after your baby is one year old.)
3. Use baby food, home-prepared food, or ground meat. Baked, broiled, or roasted meat or fish are preferred, as infants have trouble digesting bacon, sausage, and fatty or fried meats and gravy.

Recent opinion is to introduce allergic-type foods (wheat cereal and egg yolks, for example) earlier than previously recommended.[2] The reasoning behind this is to challenge the infant's immune system to minimize any future allergic reactions. However, because each infant has unique medical and family histories, it is best to check with the pediatrician before introducing such foods earlier than recommended.

Sample of a Daily Infant Feeding Plan

As mentioned, pediatricians differ widely as to when infant foods are to be introduced. Each infant acquires the developmental skills involved in eating, such as chewing and holding a cup, in his or her own time.

The following feeding plan is only a suggestion.[2] If you have any concerns about this plan, check with the pediatrician.

- Try a very small amount of the food with a new texture, and pay close attention to his or her reaction in order to prevent choking. Smaller infants likely will consume smaller amounts of formula (or number of nursing times) and food, while larger infants likely will consume greater amounts than those in the sample plan. Tune out distractions and focus on your infant's actions that communicate to you that he or she is hungry or full.
- Partial formula feeding may take place; for example, a five-month-old infant may receive three 7-ounce bottles of formula and two 3-ounce bottles, providing 27 ounces total.
- As the amount of infant food increases, the amount of formula and number of nursing times should decrease.
- When table foods are given, remove the infant's portion before adding salt, sugar, or other spices.

Formula intake should not exceed 32 ounces per day at any time—this is important. In my job as a nutrition counselor, I once evaluated the intake of an infant and discovered that the mother was giving 64 ounces of a soybean-based formula per day—twice the amount recommended for the infant's age. One of the clinic nurse's notes stated that there were open sores over the baby's body. The sores might have been caused by the excess formula intake or by the formula itself—soy can cause such an allergic response in some infants. The excess amount of formula might have overcome the infant's tolerance to the formula. I advised the mother to reduce the formula intake to 32 ounces. My second recommendation was to replace the soybean formula with another hypoallergenic formula.

For all ages mentioned, the following sample plan suggests that parents or caregivers distribute breast milk or formula and food across breakfast, midmorning, lunch, midafternoon, dinner, and bedtime. It is helpful to remember that 3 teaspoons are equal to 1 tablespoon.

You can help your infant learn to hold a cup or use a spoon by being an example, showing him or her how to do it.

Birth to One Month

At this time your infant will have acquired the mouth and tongue movements to suck and swallow liquids. When offering breast milk or formula, give the following:

- breast milk (12 times or more per day upon demand, every 90 minutes to 2 hours)
- formula (2–3 ounces per feed, every 3–4 hours, for a total of 16–21 ounces per day)

One to Two Months

- breast milk (8–10 times or more per day, upon demand, every 90 minutes to 3 hours)
- formula (3–4 ounces per feed, every 3–5 hours, for a total 21–24 ounces per day)

Two to Four Months

- breast milk (5–7 times or more/day upon demand, every 3–5 hours)
- formula (5–7 ounces/feed, every 3–5 hours, for a total 24–32 ounces/day)

Four to Six Months

At this time your infant will have acquired the mouth and tongue movements to munch and swallow commercial or homemade infant foods. Start with single-grain infant dry cereal. Offer both of the following:

- breast milk (5 times or more/day upon demand) or formula (5–7 ounces/feed, total 24–32 ounces/day)
- 1–2 tablespoons cereal (2 times per day) at age four to five months, increasing to 2–3 tablespoons (2 times per day) at age five to six months

Remember to start with 1 teaspoon of cereal mixed with breast milk or formula and gradually thicken to 1–2 tablespoons.

Six to Seven Months
At this time introduce fruits and vegetables.

- breast milk (5 times or more/day upon demand) or formula (6–8 ounces/feed, total 24–32 ounces/day)
- 1–2 tablespoons cereal (two times)
- 1–2 tablespoons vegetable, 2 tablespoons fruit, and 1 ounce juice (diluted)

Remember to start with 1 teaspoon of each new food and gradually increase the amount given.

At six months, Dr. Elizabeth Jones advises[2] introducing the use of a cup containing breast milk, formula, or juice. (Your infant will be able to hold a cup, but there will be some spillage.) In addition, if a bottle of formula is given during the night, discontinue it. Both of these feeding practices can reduce the risk of overfeeding of formula and a dependence on the bottle.

Seven to Eight Months
At this time your infant will have acquired the mouth and tongue movements to munch and swallow commercial or home-prepared meats, mashed foods, and soft foods, such as cottage cheese and plain yogurt.

- breast milk (4–5 times or more/day upon demand) or formula (6–8 ounces/feed, total 24–32 ounces/day)
- 1–2 tablespoons cereal (two times)

- 2–4 tablespoons vegetable (two times) and 2–4 tablespoons fruit, and 2 ounces juice (diluted)
- 1/2–1 tablespoon meat or fish (no shellfish), 1 mashed egg yolk mixed with breast milk or formula, and 1–2 tablespoons cottage cheese or plain yogurt (or another 1/2–1 tablespoon meat or fish)

Remember to start with 1 teaspoon of each new food and gradually increase the amount given.

Eight to Nine Months
At this time your infant will have acquired the mouth and tongue movements to chew and swallow other table foods. Introduce ground cooked meat or fish (no shellfish), soft peeled foods, soft cooked foods, mashed foods, mild cheese, and teething foods under supervision. Cereals (e.g., wheat, high-protein, mixed, and Cream of Wheat) can be introduced.

- breast milk (3–5 times or more/day upon demand); or formula (5–7 ounces/feed, total 24–32 ounces/day)
- 1–2 tablespoons cereal, half a slice of toast (cut into inch squares), and 1–2 tablespoons mashed pasta, noodles, macaroni, or rice
- 2–4 tablespoons mashed vegetable, 1–2 tablespoons mashed peeled fruit (2–3 times), and 2–3 ounces juice
- half slice mild cheese, 1–2 tablespoons ground meat or fish (or soft-cooked dried beans or peas), and 1 mashed egg yolk
- 1–2 graham cracker squares

Start with 1 teaspoon of each new food and gradually increase the amount given.

Nine to Ten Months
At this time introduce chewy finger-foods, small bite-sized pieces of soft cooked foods, and strips or slices of foods.

- breast milk (3–4 times or more/day upon demand); or formula (6–7ounces/feed, total 24–32 ounces/day)

- 1–2 tablespoons cereal and a half slice of toast (cut in inch squares)
- half of a toasted cheese sandwich (cut in inch squares)
- 2–3 tablespoons mashed vegetable (two times), 1–2 tablespoons mashed peeled fruit, 2–3 bite-sized pieces (or slices) of fruit (2 times), and 3 ounces juice
- 2 tablespoons bite-sized pieces of meat or fish, and 1–2 tablespoons cottage cheese or plain yogurt (or half slice mild cheese)
- 1–2 graham cracker squares or 1–3 low-sodium saltine crackers

Ten to Twelve Months

At this time your infant will be able to feed himself or herself (though it will be messy). Add a variety of table foods, including mild casseroles.

- breast milk (3–4 times or more/day upon demand); or formula (6–7 ounces/feed, total 24 ounces/day)
- 3–4 tablespoons cereal, half slice toast (cut in inch squares), and 1–2 tablespoons of mashed pasta, noodles, macaroni, or rice
- half a tortilla with melted cheese (cut into small parts)
- 2–4 tablespoons mashed vegetable (two times), 2–4 tablespoons mashed fruit, 3–4 bite-sized pieces of fruit (2 times), and 4 ounces juice
- 1 cooked egg yolk, 2–4 tablespoons bite-sized pieces of meat or fish, 2–3 tablespoons cottage cheese or plain yogurt (or half slice mild cheese), and 2–4 tablespoons soft cooked dried beans or peas (or another serving of meat)
- 1–2 graham crackers

Actions of Toddlers Who Express Hunger and Being Full

Once again, it is very important that mothers and fathers (or caregivers) learn to recognize their toddler's appetite-related actions of hunger and being full.

The most common actions of "being hungry" include (1) reaching out for a food or beverage or (2) pointing to a food or beverage.

The actions of being full include (1) pushing away a food or beverage, (2) playing with a food, or (3) tossing food.

Healthy Food and Beverage Intakes for Toddlers

Whole cow's milk should not be offered until after one year of age.[3] After two years of age, lower-fat milk varieties can be offered.[3]*Check with your pediatrician* before switching types of milk. At least three servings of whole or lower-fat milk should be given daily to ensure sufficient intakes of the two essential fatty acids required by toddlers.

A small child's stomach capacity is limited. Parents should offer three regular meals and two or three healthy snacks daily. Allow your toddler to determine whether and how much to eat, based upon his or her hunger. *Never force* a toddler (or infant) to take a food or to finish a food that has been offered.

Before considering the table that includes the recommended dietary intakes for toddlers, the following information will describe its contents and explain specific food groups:

- For each of the six food groups, there is a recommended number of servings to give *daily*.
- You can select from a number of food options in each of the six food groups.
- For each food option, there is a recommended amount per *serving*.
- Keeping calories in mind, select the smaller-sized fruit. Fruit pieces can include, for example, a quarter of a peeled apple or banana.
- The grain group can include small crackers, such as low-sodium saltines, or larger crackers, such as graham cracker squares.
- Fats include butter, margarine, oils, mayonnaise, salad dressing, and cream cheese—cream cheese is not a "cheese" that contributes calcium to the diet. It is basically a fat-type product.

Now refer to the "Recommended Food and Beverage Intakes for Toddlers" on the following pages regarding the number of servings and serving sizes for a one- or two-year-old. As with infants, smaller toddlers may eat less, while larger toddlers may eat more than the recommended intakes.

Recommended Food and Beverage Intakes for Toddlers
Note: 4 ounces = 1/2 cup; 4 tablespoons = 1/4 cup; 2 tablespoons = 1 ounce

Food	Serving each day	Amount of serving	Food	Serving each day	Amount of serving
Dairy	5		**Vegetables**		
Milk		4 ounces	Cooked		2–4 tablespoons
Yogurt		1/2 cup	Raw		1/4 cup
Meat and meat alternatives	2		**Grain**	6	
Meat/fish		2–4 tablespoons	Cereal		
Egg		1	Ready to eat		4 tablespoons
Cheese		Half–1 slice	Cooked		4 tablespoons
Dried beans/peas		2–4 tablespoons	Bread		Half–1 slice
Cottage cheese		2–4 tablespoons	Tortilla		Half slice
Peanut butter		1 tablespoon	Bun/bagel (1 ounce)		1/4
Fruit/ vegetables	5		Pasta/rice		2–4 tablespoons
Juice		4 ounces	Small crackers		1–3
Fruit		2–4 Tablespoons	Large crackers		1–2
Piece (small)		1/4	**Fats**	3	1 teaspoon

High-Calorie Foods in the Diets of Infants and Toddlers

Infants have an innate preference for sweet and sour tastes. Because the calories and nutrients are required for rapid growth in this first year, there is little space in the diets of infants and toddlers for high-calorie foods (high in fat and sugar or salt). For this important reason, at eight months of age, offer half a jar of infant dessert-type foods (including fruit-type) and combination dinners with gravies and sauces *no more than twice a week* for a meal or snack. Similarly, for older infants (at ten months) and toddlers who are eating table foods, offer one of the following only once or twice a week at a meal or snack:

- 2–3 vanilla wafers or 1 cream-type sandwich cookie
- 1/4 of an unfrosted brownie, piece of cake, or cupcake
- 1/4 cup of ice cream, frozen yogurt, or pudding
- 1/4 serving of other high-calorie foods, including salty snack products for toddlers
- Select those products that have less than 200 calories per serving.
- Check product label for calories per serving and serving sizes. Remember to offer only one-quarter of the serving size.

Do not offer such high-calorie sweetened beverages as fruit drinks, Kool-Aid, or soft drinks to infants or toddlers. All of these recommendations may help to sidestep sweet and salty preferences. These preferences may carry over into childhood.

Endnotes

1   C. L. Ogden et al., *Journal of the American Medical Association* 311, no. 8 (2014): 806–814.
2   E. G. Jones, *Good Nutrition for Your Baby* (San Diego: the Foundation for the Children of the Californians, 2005).
3   R. E. Kleinman, *Pediatric Nutrition Handbook* (Elk Grove, IL: American Academy of Pediatrics, 2009).

Chapter 3

Recommended Dietary Intakes for Children and Teens

Diets of American preschool and school-age children need improvement. Many youth are not meeting the US Department of Agriculture (USDA)'s recommendations for fruits and vegetables and whole-grain products.[1] Inadequate nutrients in children's diets can negatively influence their health and weight and how well they do in school. This is particularly true when meals are skipped, especially breakfast.

Because parents and caregivers are up against the unhealthy messages in the media and advertisements, as well as peer pressure that negatively influences their children and teens, they need to take action. *The most effective way to teach children healthy practices is to adopt them yourself.* Without your positive influence, unhealthy diets will continue.

Healthy Food and Beverage Intakes for Preschool Children

Based upon my experience with families having preschool children, refer to the "Recommended Food and Beverage Intakes for Preschoolers" on the following pages. Keep in mind that smaller preschoolers may eat less and larger preschoolers may eat more than the recommended intakes. Specific information about the food groups is similar to that for the "Recommended Food and Beverage Intakes for Toddlers" (chapter 2).

Recommended Food and Beverage Intakes for Preschoolers

Note: The values under each age group are the recommended amounts per serving. Also, 6 ounces = 3/4 cup, 4 tablespoons = 1/4 cup, and 2 tablespoons = 1 ounce of meat.

Food	Serv/D	Measure	2 to 3 Years	3 to 4 Years	4 to 5 Years
Dairy	3				
Milk		Ounces	6	6	6
Yogurt		Cup	1/2	1/2	1/2–3/4
Meat/Other	2				
Meat/Fish		Ounces	1–2	1–2	2
Egg		Egg	1	1	1
Cheese		Slice	1/2–1	1/2–1	1
Dried Beans/ Peas		Cup	1/4	1/4	1/4–1/2
Cottage Cheese		Cup	1/4	1/4	1/4–1/2
Peanut Butter		Tablespoons	1–2	1–2	2
Fruit/ Vegetables	5				
Juice		Ounces	4	4	4
Fruit		Cup	1/4–1/2	1/4–1/2	1/2
Piece (small)		Part of	1/4–1/2	1/4–1/2	1/2–1

Recommended Food and Beverage Intakes
for Preschoolers continued

Note: Vegetables are given as veg.

Food	Serv/D	Measure	2 to 3 Years	3 to 4 Years	4 to 5 Years
Veg					
Cooked		Cup	1/4–1/2	1/4–1/2	1/2
Raw		Cup	1/4–1/2	1/4–1/2	1/2
Grain	6				
Cereal					
Ready-to-eat		Cup	1/4–1/2	1/4–1/2	1/2–3/4
Cooked		Cup	1/4–1/2	1/4–1/2	1/2
Bread		Slice	1/2–1	1/2–1	1
Tortilla		Part of	1/2–1	1/2–1	1
Bun/Bagel (1oz)		Part of	1/4–1/2	1/4–1/2	1/2
Pasta/Rice		Cup	1/4–1/2	1/4–1/2	1/2
Small Crackers		Number of	2–3	3–4	5–6
Large Crackers		Number of	1–2	1–2	2–3
Fats	3	Teaspoon	1	1	1

High-Calorie Food and Beverages in the Diets of Preschoolers

Two or three days a week for a meal or snack, offer no more than one from each of the following:

- 3–4 vanilla wafers or 2 cream-type sandwich cookies
- half of an unfrosted brownie, piece of cake, or cupcake
- 1/2 cup of sherbet, ice cream, frozen yogurt, or pudding
- 4–6 tortilla or potato chips or 1 cup popcorn
- half a serving of other high-calorie foods (Select products that have less than 200 calories per serving.)
- Check product labels for calories per serving and serving sizes. Remember to offer only half of the serving size.

No more than two or three days a week at a meal or snack, offer 1/2 cup (4 ounces) or 1 can (6 ounces) of high-calorie (sweetened) beverages (soft drinks, fruit drinks, Kool-Aid, etc.).

Healthy Foods and Beverages for School-Age Children and Teens

As a nutrition counselor, I ask parents to recall the foods and beverages their child ate in the past twenty-four hours. In most cases, the children's diets are low in fruits and vegetables and whole-grain products. Is your child or teen eating the recommended five servings of fruits and vegetables and three servings of whole-grain products?

For dietary recommendations, refer to "Recommended Food and Beverage Intakes for School-Age Children and Teens" on the following pages. The *number of servings* and *serving sizes* are based on the USDA's Food Guide Pyramid.[1] Other recommendations not identified as the USDA's are my own. You can use these selection and preparation tips and special considerations for preschoolers as well.

Some children and teens will eat less or more than the amounts given in the recommendations, especially during the growth spurt that takes place in the teen years. Parents and caregivers should learn the recommended portion sizes to keep calories in check. As with toddlers, offer appropriate portion sizes and allow the child or teen to determine whether and how much to eat. It is very important *not to prompt* children or teens to finish eating if they are not inclined to do so.

Teach appropriate portion sizes when children begin to serve themselves. If they take too large of a serving, emphasize how important appropriate portion sizes are to the maintaining of a healthy weight. This is especially true for teens, who frequently eat larger portions at fast-food establishments or other places outside of the home. Assure your children, tots to teens, that they can have more if they still feel hungry. If second helpings are desired, begin with small amounts, starting with a tablespoon at a time.

In present-day society, where supersizes are purchased without question, it is very important to strike a balance between placing boundaries around food intake and calories (portion sizes), while encouraging your child's self-reliance on feelings of hunger and being full.

In the educational classes at the health department, we used plastic food models to teach appropriate portion sizes. One day, I left the models in the classroom. Upon returning, I found that some were missing. Who had swiped the plastic food? Later, we discovered that an elderly person from the adjoining county nursing home had found a way into the classroom, selected the plastic foods of choice, and had taken them. The lesson here is that it is never too late to learn appropriate portion sizes.

Importance of Eating Healthy

For optimum bone growth, three servings of milk or other dairy products are recommended daily for children, nine years old through teens. Getting calcium from dairy products is related to healthier weights.[2] From tots to teens, strive to include five or more servings of fruits and vegetables, including a vitamin C–rich source and vitamin A–rich source daily (or at least three times weekly). It's also recommended to eat several whole-grain products daily.

When we eat food, our bodies produce oxidants, which cause damage to cell membranes (arteries) and DNA. Such damage increases our risk for heart disease, stroke, and cancer. Powerful antioxidants are present in both fruits and vegetables (vitamins A and C) and whole-grain products (vitamin E and the mineral selenium). A number of other protective substances also are found in fruits and vegetables. These antioxidants work hard to minimize such oxidative damage. It is up to us to take advantage of these preventive plant constituents offered by nature.

Recommended Food and Beverage Intakes
for School-Age Children and Teens

Dairy Products

- Two or three servings daily of dairy products are recommended for children 5–8 years old; three servings daily for children 9–12 years old and teens.
- Select fat-free or low-fat (1 percent) products.

One serving is 8 ounces (1 cup) of milk or 6–8 ounces (3/4 or 1 cup) of yogurt.[1] If 2 percent milk is preferred, count it as two servings of milk *plus* one serving of fat in the dietary plan. The third serving can be 2 ounces of cheese, considered here as a meat alternative.

Meat and Meat Alternatives

- Both select (lean) cuts and choice (some fat) cuts of meat are included, a combination of meats quite often consumed by many families.
- As often as possible, it is best to choose lean cuts of meat, lean hamburger, and low-fat luncheon meats, hot dogs, cheese, and peanut butter.
- For meats, determine that amount after cooking and after removing bones, skin, and fat from the edges of meat. A 4-ounce piece of raw meat will yield 3 ounces of cooked meat.
- Two or three servings are recommended daily (a total of 5–7 ounces).[1]
- An average portion of meat and an alternative is 2 or 3 ounces.[1] This could include one of the following:[1]

  2–3 ounces of poultry, meat, or fish
  2–3 ounces of sandwich meats

> 2 ounces (1/4 cup) of tuna (water-packed or drained of oil)
> 2–3 ounces of cheese

An ounce of meat or an alternative can include one of the following:[1]

> 1 hot dog or 1 egg
> 1 tablespoon of peanut butter
> 1/2 cup of dried beans or peas

Consider the size of a 3-ounce patty, stack of thin slices, or a piece of meat as being four inches by three inches and a half inch thick. Examples include half a chicken breast; a regular-sized hamburger, tenderloin, or pork chop; or a chicken or fish fillet.

In addition, consider a chicken wing as 1 ounce and the leg and thigh as 2 ounces.

Two ounces of cheese is two thin slices or the size of a two-inch square chunk.

When meat and meat alternatives with a higher fat content are consumed, count this as one serving of the following plus one serving of fat in the dietary plan:

- each ounce of prime cuts
- each ounce of other meats high in fat (meatloaf, ground beef, bacon, etc.)
- each ounce of sandwich meats (bologna, pastrami) and 1 hot dog
- each ounce of American, Swiss, cheddar, jack, mozzarella cheese or other chesses
- each ounce of fried chicken or fish
- each egg scrambled or fried
- each tablespoon of peanut butter

Because of the high fat content, whether it's one, two, or three ounces or tablespoons, consume only one or two of such foods no more than twice weekly.

Prepare by baking, grilling, or broiling. Fry only occasionally.

Fruits and Vegetables

Five or more servings of fruits and vegetables are recommended daily.[1] One serving is equal to the following:[1]

- 4 ounces juice
- one small piece of fruit
- 1/2 cup berries or other fruits
- 1 cup melon
- 1/4 cup dried fruits

One serving of vegetables is equal to the following:[1]

- 1/2 cup cooked vegetables
- 1/2 cup chopped raw vegetables or sticks
- 1 cup leafy raw vegetables (lettuce or spinach)
- 3/4 cup vegetable juice.

Quite often, children and teens prefer corn and potatoes, especially french fries, which have a higher fat content. Count each small serving or package of french fries as one serving of vegetable *plus* one serving of fat in the dietary plan.

Such vegetables as corn, potatoes, peas, and lima beans contain a higher carbohydrate content. Because of this, it is best to offer these vegetables at mealtime only three or four days a week. Work hard to encourage your children or teens to consume a wide variety of vegetables, especially the colorful vegetables, by repeatedly offering them over time. Colorful vegetables (for example, red, deep yellow or orange, or green) have a higher content of vitamins and minerals and protective substances that can keep your family healthy.

You may wish to offer a colorful vegetable plus a serving of a whole-grain pasta or wild rice. Fresh, frozen, and canned vegetables may be selected (although canned vegetables have a higher salt content), but avoid fruits canned in heavy syrup.

Breads, Cereals, and Pastas (Grains)

Six or more servings of grains are recommended daily.[1] One serving (preferably whole grain) is equal to the following:[1]

- slice of bread or small roll
- 1/2 hamburger or hot dog bun
- 1/2 small bagel (1 ounce) or 1/2 english muffin
- 5–6 small or 3–4 large crackers
- 1/2 cup cooked cereal, rice, or pasta
- 3/4 cup (1 ounce) of ready-to-eat cereal (lower added sugar preferred)

A small biscuit or muffin may be eaten occasionally. Among the six servings, strive to include three or more whole-grain products. Gradually introduce whole-grain products—eating too much at one time can cause digestive upset. This also may apply to too many fruits and vegetables.

Fats and Oils

Two or more servings of fats and oils are recommended daily.[1] One serving is equal to the following:[1]

- 1 teaspoon margarine, butter, mayonnaise, or vegetable oil
- 1 tablespoon salad dressing, cream cheese, or sour cream

Select fat-free, low-fat, reduced-fat, or light products.

Other Foods and Beverages

Some foods and beverages contain very few calories; that is, less than 25 calories per servings. Such foods and beverages can be included in diet without considering them in the total daily intake of calories. These include condiments, such as mustard and ketchup; coffee, tea, or diet soft drinks; and certain fat-free products. Check product labels for calories per serving and serving size.

Special Considerations

The following recommendations can be applied to foods and beverages that are prepared at home or at restaurants, fast-food establishments, or delis or that are commercially frozen or canned products.

How can dishes containing a number of ingredients (such as casseroles, chili, soups) be included in a dietary plan? If homemade, divide the measured amount of each ingredient by the number of servings that the recipe suggests. Consider only those ingredients that contribute the most to the recipe. For such dishes, a recommended serving is 1 cup. For example, 1 cup of macaroni and cheese or a tuna casserole may contain about 3/4 cup of noodles and 1 ounce of tuna or cheese. Count this dish as having two servings from the grain group and one serving from the meat group.

Keep in mind that uncooked pasta doubles in size when cooked; for example, 1 cup uncooked becomes 2 cups cooked. For similar commercially prepared dishes, do your best to determine the amount of each ingredient. Check product labels for number of servings per container and serving size.

Likewise, for commercial meals and products (such as pizzas, tacos, hamburgers) determine the amount of each component. For example, a cheeseburger would contain one bun (two servings from the grain group); 3 ounces of hamburger, and 1 ounce of cheese (four servings from the meat group). Mustard, ketchup, and pickles are "free."

Count a meal of 3 ounces of turkey, 1/2 cup dressing, and 1/2 cup green beans, as three servings of meat, one serving of grains, and one serving of vegetables.

High-Calorie Foods and Beverages in the Diets of School-Age Children and Teens

Reduce the intake of high-calorie foods (high in fat, sweetened-type foods, and salty snack products, including sweets, desserts, and pastries) to one serving at one meal or snack, no more than three or four days a week for school-age children and teens. Check product labels for calories per serving and serving sizes.

Reduce intake of high-calorie sweetened beverages (including soft drinks) to no more than one cup (8 ounces) or can (12 ounces) for teens, three or four days weekly; and one cup or can for school-age children, two or three days weekly.

Vitamins and Mineral Supplements

Healthy children and teens who consume nourishing meals and snacks do not require a vitamin and/or mineral supplement. If you give a supplement, however, intakes from dietary sources, fortified foods, and the supplement should not exceed 100 percent of a vitamin's or mineral's recommended level. Check supplement labels. For healthy children and teens who are on nutritionally balanced diets, consuming more than the recommended daily allowance (RDA) of vitamins and minerals does not provide additional health benefits. The idea that one tablet is good, so two or more may be better is not valid. Excess can result in toxicity or unhealthy interactions between the supplement and other vitamins or minerals and prescribed medications.

Remember that vitamins and minerals from supplements are not as effective in preventing disease as those acquired from food. Fruits and vegetables and whole-grain products also have many protective substances that fight against disease.

Often, a physician may recommend a vitamin and/or mineral supplement if there is a medical problem, like anemia, or an eating problem, like anorexia. In such cases, the amount of the vitamin or mineral may be higher than the recommended level when under medical supervision.

The functions and sources of certain vitamins and minerals are briefly discussed here:

Vitamin A is important for healthy vision and tissue. Vitamin A in the form of beta carotene occurs in dark-green leafy vegetables and deep yellow (or orange) fruits and vegetables. Such vegetables include broccoli, spinach, greens, carrots, and sweet potatoes. Fruits include cantaloupe, peaches, and apricots. Beta carotene is converted to vitamin A in the body.

Vitamin C is important in wound healing and acts as an antioxidant, which prevents damage to cells. It is found in citrus fruits and juices (such as orange and grapefruit), in melons (such as cantaloupe), and in berries (such as strawberries). Vegetables with vitamin C include green peppers, broccoli, brussels sprouts, cauliflower, tomatoes, and cabbage.

Folic acid (or folate) is important for healthy cells and DNA, and it plays a significant role in many chemical reactions in the body. Research has shown that folate can help reduce the risk of giving birth to an infant with neural tube defects (spinal defects). Folate is present in dark-green leafy vegetables, such as broccoli and spinach, and orange juice. It is also found in fortified cereals and grains.

Iron is important for healthy red blood cells, which carry oxygen to tissues. Iron is present in whole-grain, enriched bread, and cereal products. Iron occurs in dried fruits, such as raisins and prunes, and such vegetables as spinach and greens. When such foods are eaten along with a rich vitamin C source, absorption of iron is increased. Meat is a good source of iron because this iron is readily absorbed.

Calcium is necessary for healthy teeth and bones. The best sources of calcium in the diet are milk and milk products. Calcium also has been added to some juices, candies, and calcium-fortified cereals. Check labels.

Endnotes

1   "Food Guide Pyramid: A Guide to Daily Food Choices," *Home and Garden Bulletin*, no. 572 (Washington, DC: US Dept of Agriculture, Human Nutrition Information Service, 1992.)
2   M. A. Pereira et al., "Dairy consumption, obesity, and Insulin Resistance Syndrome in young adults: The CARDIA study," *J Am Med Assoc* 287 (2002): 2081–2089.

Chapter 4

Parenting and Promoting Healthy Eating Practices

During the early years of life when eating practices are being established, encourage your children to explore new foods and beverages, and allow independence in food selections. Here, you may wish to take the advice of pediatric experts who recommend, "Offer healthy options."[1] "Parents can ask the child to choose between an apple or banana for a snack, not an apple or a cookie."[1] This practice will help healthy foods become familiar to children—remember that children will eat food that has become familiar to them. As children become older, have them take their own portion sizes. Encourage children and teens to respond to their feelings of hunger and being full. Praise them when they do so.

All of the above recommendations help strike a balance between the child's and teen's need for independence and a parent's need to teach healthy ways of eating. Doing so will reduce conflicts between parents and children at meal times.

Unhealthy Parental Feeding Practices

There are certain unhealthy feeding practices that I have learned through my experience and those of Birch and Fisher, experts in child development, including that out of a weight-related concern for a child or teen, parents may become "controlling"[2] or overly demanding (such as telling the child, "Eat what is left on your plate") or "restrictive."[2] They may forbid high-calorie foods and beverages, such as cookies and Kool-Aid. It is best to check with your child's physician before making any significant dietary changes.

In addition, the following feeding practices definitely are "do nots":

- *Do not* offer high-calorie foods and beverages as a reward or for comfort.
- *Do not* deny high-calorie foods as a punishment.
- *Do not* promise a sweet or favorite food in order to get the child to finish a meal or parent-preferred food.

Do reward positive food-related behaviors with praise, compliments, special attention, or a favorite activity.

Remember that unwise parental feeding practices can interfere with a child's ability to regulate his or her intake. Because of this, when given the opportunity, children will overeat on high-calorie foods and beverages because they are highly flavorful and, in many cases, readily available. This results in extra calories and an undesirable weight gain. The ultimate goal is to teach your children and teens how to select, prepare, and enjoy *balanced* meals and snacks that provide a variety of all foods and beverages in appropriate amounts, as well as how often they should eat.

Making Healthy Eating a Family Affair

Increasing the number of times you share meals as a family weekly and reducing the amount of screen time daily by children are two effective measures to help reduce the rising rate of obesity among our children and teens.

Important benefits associated with eating meals together as a family include the following:

- Nutritional
  Parents have the opportunity to prepare nourishing meals at home. Carry-out or fast-food meals are higher in calories, sugar, fat, cholesterol, and sodium.

- Educational
  Parents can teach and model appropriate eating skills and mealtime etiquette; children can learn and practice such skills and etiquette.

- Social
  Family meals can provide a special time for sharing of positive experiences, new ideas, daily events, local and world news, and future plans.

- Emotional
  Parents and siblings can offer a caring environment in which emotional concerns and problems can be aired and possible solutions discussed. (Postpone discussing problems related to discipline or arguments for a later time.)

I would recommend having a family meal five or more times each week. Be firm that children and teens meet this family goal. I would also advise that when you are setting healthy goals for your family (chapter 9), select family meals as an initial goal.

A friend and I have discussed the importance of family meals. Although she works full time, she tries to fix a balanced meal for most dinners. She mentioned that when her son Nicholas invited a friend to dinner, the friend couldn't believe the meal she served. He said, "You eat like this every night?" Many of Nicholas's friends are surprised by the array of healthy foods that Nicholas brings to school for his lunch. It makes me wonder how often some of today's children have a balanced meal.

Learn to prepare easy-to-fix, nourishing meals and snacks. Add variety by taking your family meal to a local park, beach, lake, or even out to your backyard. Share family meals with neighbors by having a potluck or barbeque.

Family sharing a meal together

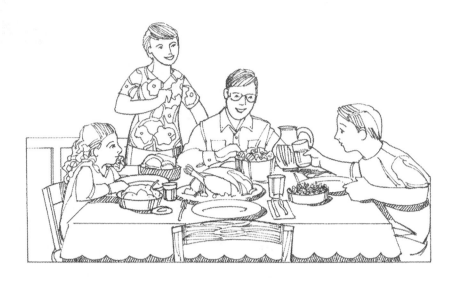

The Importance of Reducing Television Viewing During Meals and Snacks

Watching television while eating a meal can result in overeating and undesirable weight gain, as children and adults may lose track of how much they are eating.

The American Academy of Pediatrics recommends that parents "limit children's total media time (with entertainment media) to no more than 1 to 2 hours of quality programming per day."[3] I believe that computer time (for purposes other than homework) should be included within this two-hour limitation as well. Allow extra time for homework if needed. The American Academy of Pediatrics also suggests that "Discourage television viewing for children younger than 2 years."[3] In a recent news report, pediatricians also caution parents not to give computer tablets to these younger children as well. *It is best* that children and teens watch television and use computers in the family areas of the home.

Why should you limit television and computer time? These modern electronics replace the time that children could devote to physical activity and using their imaginations for creative play. I remember as kids we would raid our mom's cabinet for canned foods and play grocery store under the kitchen table.

I would recommend the following practical pointers to help mothers and fathers:

- Keep a weekly log of daily activities for each child and teen.
- Note how many hours are devoted to television and computer use for entertainment and school purposes.
- Also, record any food or beverages consumed at these times.
- To be effective, steps to gradually reduce any excess TV or computer time are described in chapter 6, and steps to reduce the frequency of food and beverage eaten during these times are described in chapter 5.
- Mothers and fathers should work with their child or teen to select age-appropriate programs or video games for the two hours. This can prevent an all-out rebellion.
- In addition, have your child or teen create a list of physical activities that can replace the times of inactivity, especially when food and beverages are being consumed.

In my time, kids would hide under their bed covers at night to read a book with a flashlight. In today's world, kids are more likely to hide under the covers with a computer tablet and a favorite snack. Another suggestion for parents is to make unannounced visits on different days and at different times during the early night hours.

Meals and Snacks for Children

One summer I was asked to evaluate a preschool program. Many of its practices are applicable to the feeding of preschool and school-age children, and I would like to share them with you here.

Remember that breakfast is important for children. Skipping breakfast (or any meal) can negatively affect a child, both physically and mentally. I strongly suggest that at least one parent or a caregiver be at all meals. This can ensure that children are present and are eating healthy foods and beverages.

Because children—younger ones in particular—need to eat more frequently, offer three equally spaced regular meals and two or three snacks daily. For example, breakfast, lunch, and dinner; midmorning, afternoon, and evening snacks. Do not allow eating or drinking of anything but water (especially not high-calorie foods and beverages) during nonmeal and nonsnack times. This can prevent excessive snacking that can add extra calories and weight.

As for a family meal, try to prepare each meal and snack in an attractive way by including various shapes, textures, flavors, and especially colors. (Choose at least two of those four.)

Fixing nourishing meals can be simple. Include a protein from the meat group and/or a dairy product, a fruit and/or vegetable, and a selection from the grain group. For example, have a peanut butter sandwich (protein and grain), carrot sticks (vegetable), apple (fruit), and milk (dairy). For variety in the meal and to encourage children to accept new foods, offer a new food along with familiar ones. If your child is reluctant to accept the new food, tell him or her to take just a bite or two.

Everyone at the table should eat the same foods that have been prepared; that is, don't prepare favorite foods for a specific child or teen. Snack times are the best opportunity for individual eating preferences. Most children, especially the young ones, prefer foods prepared separately rather than in combined dishes, such as casseroles. They generally enjoy finger foods, such as carrot and celery sticks, cheese cubes, or pieces of fruit, which make excellent snacks.

Carefully plan meals and snacks so that they are not rushed—a common occurrence due to busy schedules. In addition, provide a comfortable and quiet eating environment. To prevent a struggle at the table with a child who is cranky or tired, try for a nap prior to the meal or snack. Alternately, read to your child from a favorite book or play a favorite card game for ten or fifteen minutes, or have an older sibling do so.

If arguing or squabbles occurs between siblings at the table, ask the children to leave the table. Turn off radios and televisions, and don't allow cell phones, computers, or iPods at the table.

It's also important to teach your children and teens how to politely refuse food when grandparents, other relatives, or friends pressure them to eat. For example, a grandmother may say, "Have another slice of my chocolate cake."

Begin teaching your child the above eating practices in his or her early years and reinforce the practices as he or she grows older.

In today's society, many mothers work full- or part-time, and many preschoolers eat some of their meals and snacks at day care centers. Find out the types of meals and snacks the center offers, and strongly request healthy meals and snacks if the center is not already providing them, as well as a variety of physical activities.

Acquire weekly menus from your child's or teen's school or day care center. This will help you to plan dinners and snacks for a better nutritional balance of nutrients and calories. In addition, prepare nourishing school lunches so that your child doesn't need to rely on school snack-bar selections, which often are high in calories, fat, and sugar and are eaten in large portions.

Many American families struggle financially and may believe that offering a variety of foods and beverages is impossible. There are ways to stay within your budget, however, and still provide nourishing food. For example, some farmers markets accept the Link card and offer discounts to families with limited income. If possible, buy extra produce in the summer to freeze for winter months. (Check with your local health department's Cooperative Extension Service for tips on freezing and canning of produce.)

In addition, check with your local health department's special supplemental nutrition program for Women, Infants, and Children (WIC). If your family meets financial guidelines, you can receive such grocery items as formula, milk, eggs, and other healthy food and beverages. Vouchers for such grocery items are given to expectant and breast-feeding mothers, infants, and children up to five years of age. Another helpful resource is the book *Using Coupons: Encouraging Hope* by Kimberly McCormick, available at www.amazon.com. Grocery money that is saved by coupons can be used elsewhere.

Meals and Snacks for Teens

Many teens have a busy and hectic life. Because they frequently eat on the run, they may purchase larger portions of high-calorie foods and beverages from fast-food establishments. Teens also are notorious for skipping meals, especially breakfast.

Sit down with your family members and set priorities, the first of which should be to *establish a healthy schedule by reducing the number of activities*.

- In addition to school requirements, religious activities and part-time job commitments, teens should choose only one or two extracurricular activities.
- For example, one activity may be school-related, such as playing sports on the high school team, and the other may not be school-related, such as attending a club meeting.

The second priority should be to *acquire healthier eating practices* such as the following:

- Strongly discourage skipping meals (especially breakfast) and continuous snacking throughout the day. Encourage instead having regular mealtimes and snack times.
- Share with your teen the important benefits of family meals. Even if your teen works part-time while going to school, have him or her join you as often as possible in family meals.
- Have him or her take a healthy lunch to school at least three times weekly.
- To help reduce the amount of high-calorie foods and beverages your teen eats and drinks, he or she should keep a log of such foods and beverages purchased at fast-food restaurants and at school to easily see those that are purchased most frequently. He or she then can visit the fast-food websites to check the calorie content of the foods and beverages purchased. This will help your teen realize how "calorie-expensive" such foods are.
- Try to encourage your teen to find the healthier alternatives on the fast-food websites. Use the same healthier alternatives to replace the unhealthy ones purchased at school.

The third priority is to *acquire healthier activities*. Strongly encourage your teens to replace one hour of television or recreational computer time with a moderate-intensity physical activity, such as briskly walking, swimming, or running. Doing these activities with another family member can help your teen keep these activities as a priority. Also encourage your teen to participate in family-centered activities, such as biking, hiking, and swimming together.

Emphasize that the above recommendations will help your teen obtain optimum growth and health and, if needed, a better weight during the adolescent growth spurt when nutrient demands are high.

Participating in Family Responsibilities Related to Meals and Snacks

Involve children and teens in the following: (1) planning healthy meals and snacks, (2) creating grocery lists for meals and snacks, (3) searching for coupons for healthy foods and beverages, (4) comparison shopping using nutrition labeling, (5) fixing healthy meals and snacks, and (6) preparing recipes and finding new ones.

Children and teens are more likely to eat or taste what they prepare themselves. In addition, have the family plan, plant, and take care of a vegetable garden to encourage your children to taste different vegetables and learn their nutritional value. Encourage your child to participate in any school or community activities that can add to the six skills mentioned above. For example, when there is a school fund-raiser involving commercial food products, discuss those products that would be the healthiest choices and why. Also, you may have your child or teen prepare a family recipe for a church potluck.

My mother and I shared a love of cooking. Some of my favorite memories as a teen include preparing new recipes with my mother, one of which was cream puffs. We knew that if pie crust dough is handled too much, it becomes tough; we thought the same applied to cream puff dough, and so we were careful with it. Still, the cream puffs came out of the oven as hard as rocks.

Later, I learned in one of my food classes at the university that cream puff dough should be mixed or beaten until it has a shiny or satin look. This look indicates that enough air bubbles have been forced into the dough to allow it to rise in the oven.

Upon rising, a hollow pocket and a defined cap result. The next step is to carefully remove the "cap," fill the pocket with pudding (sugar-free recommended), and replace the cap. An optional step is to lightly dust the cream puffs with powdered sugar. These puffy delights can be a special treat for your family.

When your child tries to create new recipes, he or she likely will make a few mistakes but should try to learn from this experience and continue to explore new recipes. Remember that preparing recipes is a valuable experience; it helps your child to learn the specific amounts of ingredients that represent everyday household measurements. For example, your child can see how much cooked cereal is present in a half cup and how much sugar is present in a teaspoon. These household measurements that are the portion sizes given in all the dietary recommendations presented in this book.

Children preparing a healthy recipe

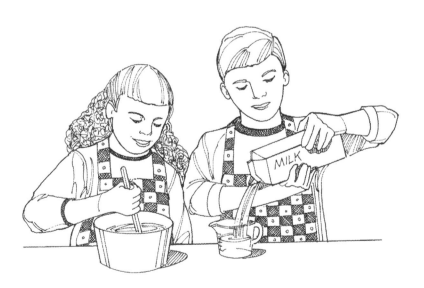

Teaching Your Children and Teens about Nutrition Labels

1. Commercial product labels list nutrition information beginning with a list of the ingredients in descending amounts, with the highest amount listed first.

Because monounsaturated, and omega-3 fats are healthy fats, select products that list those fats and oils first; for example, canola, olive, and peanut oils (monounsaturated fats); and fish such as tuna and fish oils (omega-3 fats).

Saturated fats and trans-fats are unhealthy. Avoid selecting products for which the *first ingredients* are saturated fats (butter or lard) or partially hydrogenated fats, which are high in trans-fats. Trans-fats are artificially produced when vegetable oils are hydrogenated in order to give them a more solid consistency. Select soft margarines instead of stick margarines because they contain fewer trans-fats.

Products that have sugar as one of the first three or four ingredients should be considered as having a high sugar content.

2. Look for special labeling.

Families need to watch the amount of fat in their diets. For each gram of protein or carbohydrate eaten, the body produces four calories of energy, whereas for each gram of fat, nine calories are produced—that's more than twice as many. Look for labels with lowering degrees of fat, starting with fat-free, then low-fat, and then reduced-fat. If a product is "light," it has a reduced number of calories.

3. Read the nutrition facts panel.

Try to compare products with similar serving sizes. It is easier to compare percentages of the recommended levels of vitamins and minerals in the product when both products have a serving size of a half cup, rather than one product having a serving size of a half cup and the other a serving size of one cup. Be careful because some packages or containers have more than one serving. Compare products for the following *per serving*:
- lower calories
- lower total fat
- higher percent of recommended levels of vitamins and minerals
- higher fiber content
- lower cholesterol content
- lower sodium content

You will begin to notice that the format of some labels have been changed. Product manufacturers need to replace present labeling information with new labeling requirements by July of 2018.

Endnotes

1   S. E. Barlow and W. H. Dietz, "Obesity evaluation and treatment: Expert committee recommendations" *Pediatrics* 102 (1998): 1–11.
2   L. L. Birch and J. O. Fisher, "Development of eating behaviors among children and adolescents" *Pediatrics* 101 (1998): 539–549.
3   American Academy of Pediatrics, Committee on Public Education. "Children, adolescents and television." *Pediatrics* 107 (2001): 423-426.

Chapter 5

Parenting and Correcting Unhealthy Feeding Practices

Why are millions of US children and teens overweight or obese? Excess weight results from an imbalance in the body's energy equation. This energy equation consists of energy intake (calories taken in) and energy (calories) expended, which is necessary to sustain life and for physical activity. Many American children and teens are eating too many calories and expending too few calories. This difference in calories, over time, can result in an unhealthy weight gain.

Children have the "ability to regulate intake."[1] That is, children are able to maintain a healthy weight because they are able to control how much they eat. However, such control can be overridden by unwise practices by parents or caregivers, like forcing children to clean their plates and forbidding them to eat foods high in fat and sugar, and by present-day eating practices, described below. Children are constantly bombarded by unhealthy media messages that encourage the consumption of nutrient-poor foods and beverages. The primary unhealthy eating practices that have contributed to weight gain include the following:

- eating larger portions
- eating foods that are high in fat, sugar, and salt
- drinking high-calorie (or sweetened) beverages
- eating more meals and snacks outside the home
- eating fewer meals with the family

Another important factor is the physical inactivity of many American children and teens. Without the positive influence of parents or caregivers, unhealthy eating practices and physical inactivity will continue.

The best way to combat obesity is to prevent it. As children become older, they also become more resistant to change. This is why healthy eating and physical activity need to be established early in life.

Positive Examples by Parents, Caregivers, and Older Brothers and Sisters

Your eating practices do shape those of your children in significant ways. The powerful influence of an adult example cannot be overemphasized. If parents or caregivers eat large portions, eat at a rapid pace, or overeat high-calorie foods and beverages, they cannot expect children to do differently.

Positive eating practices, established in the early years, not only benefit the child, but then he or she can become a positive role model to a younger sibling. Children look up to their older brothers and sisters and will adopt their eating practices as well. By instilling positive practices that can be strengthened throughout life, your children will be less likely to be influenced by peer pressure for unhealthy preferences and practices. This is also true when children confront the ever-present magnetic appeal of certain foods due to the marketing strategies from the media.

Recommended Frequency of Eating Practices

The recommended frequency (number of days per week) is based upon the nutrition principle of moderation (how often). This recommended frequency is designed to strike a balance between being too flexible and too controlling with regard to your family's eating practices. Undoubtedly, this frequency will require significant changes for some families, but the best approach is to make small changes over time.

The following practical advice will help mothers, fathers, and other caregivers to confront and correct the major unhealthy eating practices that have given rise to the obesity problem among our children and teens.

Eating Regular Meals and Snacks

Problem

When eating on the run, you are more likely to select fast-food or convenience items with high-calorie value (highly sweet or high in fat).

Recommendations

It would be better to pace your day in order to prepare regular nourishing meals and snacks. *Strive to have family members eat regular meals and snacks every day*. If you are rushed, however, make a conscious effort to select the healthier fast-food or convenience item. Try to prepare healthy lunches for work or school on three or more days a week—and remind your children not to "swap" their lunches with other children.

Becoming Tuned In to Your Internal Feelings of Hunger and Being Full

Problem

Impulsive and *erratic* eating should be avoided, as these can lead to overeating of less nourishing meals and snacks.

Recommendations

Ideally, the best approach is to rely on your internal feelings of hunger and being full to control your eating. Responding only to internal feelings is an effective way to control food intake, as it reduces the risk of impulsive or erratic eating due to stress, boredom, or strong emotions (anger, frustration, depression, etc.).

Also, resist responding to such external cues as TV or advertisements about food, as well as the desire or pressure to start or stop eating just because others do. Relying solely on internal feelings, however, is difficult for many individuals. Consider the following: when the fuel gauge in a car is on empty, the driver knows that there is a need for gas to power the engine. Similarly, an empty stomach indicates to your brain that there is a need for food and the calories it provides to power your body.

Your stomach is your "energy gauge." There are several degrees of "being empty" or needing calories.

- The levels of hunger that indicate the need for calories are represented by values ranging from -1 (slightly hungry) to -3 (very hungry).
- The state of being no longer hungry but not yet full is represented by a reading of 00.
- When calories are received, the levels of fullness are represented by values ranging from +1 (slightly full) to +3 (very full).

Work hard to have family members respond to feelings of hunger and being full at meals and snacks.

Your Energy Gauge

- +3; very full (Avoid this level. If it occurs, take a leisurely walk.)
- +2; full (Stop eating.)
- +1; slightly full (Continue eating.)
- 00; no longer hungry but not yet full (Continue eating.)
- -1; slightly hungry (Continue eating or start eating lightly.)
- -2; hungry (Continue eating or start eating moderately.)
- -3; very hungry (Avoid this level. If it occurs, eat slowly and moderately at a steady pace.)
- Eating "lightly" could mean reducing the amount of food and number of beverages normally eaten at a given meal or snack or eating only half portions of the food and beverages normally consumed.
- Eating "moderately" could mean consuming the food and beverages normally eaten at a given meal or snack in appropriate portion (or serving) sizes and taking a second serving only if you feel hungry.

It is important to encourage your family members to become more sensitive to their internal feelings of hunger and satiety—the earlier, the better.

Help your older children use "Your Energy Gauge." For younger children, have them place their hands over their stomachs and ask them, "Is your tummy full?"

The concept of Your Energy Gauge is related to the "Blastoff" game, an interactive computer game that helps children and teens learn to make healthy dietary choices. They are asked to select from different foods and beverages for each meal and snack in order to reach "Planet Power" by fueling their rocket with energy (or calories) for the day. Calories based on these meals are entered into a fuel tank that determines whether or not the calories are in excess of the children's needs. Put your children in the pilot's seat at www.usda. gov/mypyramidforkids and click on "Blastoff" game.

Reducing Your Portion Sizes

Problem

Many restaurants offer larger portion sizes, such as "supersize" sandwiches, fries, or beverages. Because of widespread and persuasive advertising, such products are accepted and purchased *without question*.

Recommendations

- It is very important, however, to pass on such products and select the regular or smaller-sized meals and drinks.
- In addition, pay close attention to the recommended portion (serving) sizes on commercial product labels, and replace larger dinner plates, soup and cereal bowls, and tumblers and mugs with smaller ones.
- Remember to offer an appropriate portion size and then allow your child a second helping (start with a tablespoonful) if he or she is still hungry.

Gradually incorporate these ideas in small steps into your everyday routines, and work hard to have family members eat appropriate portion sizes for each meal and snack.

Parents need to work patiently with their children (including teenagers) to correct any excessive or insufficient amounts of food consumed. Learning appropriate portion sizes at home will help safeguard your children against the ever-present allure of larger portion sizes offered outside the home.

Reducing Your Pace of Eating

Problem

A fast pace of eating can result in eating too much and gaining unwanted pounds.

Recommendations

Major meals (such as lunch and dinner) should last between twenty and thirty minutes. At the same time, focus on what your internal feelings are telling you. To help you slow your pace of eating, remember the following:

- Take smaller bites and chew each bite thoroughly.
- Periodically set down your fork or spoon between bites.
- Pause for a few minutes throughout the meal.

Teach children and teens these simple measures to reduce the pace of eating as well.

Reducing Your Intake of High-Calorie Foods

Problem

Nutrient-rich products—low-fat dairy items; lean meats, fish, and poultry; whole grains; and fruits and vegetables—are low in fat and high in protein. High-calorie or nutrient-poor products are high in fat and salt (e.g., chips, pretzels) or high in fat and sugar (pastries, desserts, and other sweets). Such products are often referred to as empty-calorie foods because of their lower nutrient content.

Because nutrient-rich foods have a higher protein, fiber, and water content, and because they are digested and absorbed more slowly, these foods have the ability to delay hunger.

Because high-calorie products are highly flavorful and readily available, adults and children alike quite often consume excessive amounts of such products, adding extra weight over time. This can place them on the path to obesity.

High-calorie products do add variety and pleasure to everyday meals and snacks.

Recommendations

Keep in mind that all types of food and beverages, in appropriate amounts, can fit into a nutritionally balanced diet. Appropriate portion sizes and moderation (how often eaten) are key in keeping the calories in high-calorie foods within reasonable limits. *Do not* tell your children that some foods *should* be eaten and others *should not*.

The best approach is to watch carefully the amount of high-calorie foods eaten early in life (chapter 1), especially for children with a strong family history of obesity.

The following practical pointers may be helpful:

- Do not consistently replace nutrient-rich food with high-calorie food.
- *If your family eats a relatively healthy diet, allow a high-calorie food (in an appropriate amount) at one meal or snack, but no more than three or four days a week for adults, teens, and school-age children.*
- *Preschool children should have half of a serving no more than two or three days a week.*
- *Infants and toddlers should have a quarter serving no more than one or two days a week.*

- You may wish to review the description of high-calorie foods for infants and toddlers in chapter 2 and for preschoolers in chapter 3.
- Check product labels for calories per serving and recommended serving sizes. You may wish to make a list of the serving sizes on favorite products, just in case you desire to make them from scratch.

If your family is consuming too many high-calorie products, gradually replace them with nutrient-rich foods until the above-recommended frequency is acquired. Slowly reduce the purchase of the nutrient-poor products, and then store those purchased items out of reach. To reduce the temptation to overeat, place such products in small containers (such as small baggies, custard cups, or eight-ounce margarine tubs).

Keep in mind that *both* healthy eating and exercise can overcome the overeating of highly tempting, flavorful high-calorie foods. Such foods could rob you and your children of a healthy weight or prevent you from acquiring one.

Reducing Your Intake of High-Calorie Beverages

Problem

High-calorie sweetened beverages, including regular soft drinks, fruit drinks, and Kool-Aid, can be considered nutrient-poor products. High fructose corn syrup (HFCS), which contains both fructose and glucose, is used in most soft drinks. Check the list of ingredients on product labels of sweetened beverages and other commercial products for HFCS.

Coffee and tea that are highly sweetened (more than one teaspoon) with table sugar or honey are considered high-calorie beverages.

Popular soft drinks have an average of 160 calories per can.

Table sugar (sucrose) contains fructose, which is bonded to glucose. During digestion, however, the bonds are broken, giving rise to a mixture of fructose and glucose, like that found in HFCS. Thus, one serving of an HFCS soft drink would contain the equivalent of eight teaspoons of sugar per can. Just think about how many calories and the amount of sugar you would drink with two or three servings.

Recommendations

The American Heart Association (www.americanheartassociation.org) advises no more than nine teaspoons of sugar daily. As additional caution, both fructose and glucose cause dental decay.

Adults and children would benefit from reducing their intake of soft drinks and other sweetened beverages. I strongly recommend that you do not consistently (to a great extent) replace nutrient-rich beverages with nutrient-poor ones and that you try to replace soft drinks and other sweetened beverages with water or juice.

- *Adults who prefer sweetened beverages should consume no more than one cup (eight ounces) or one can (twelve ounces) daily.*
- *For teens, no more than one cup or one can, three or four days weekly.*
- *For school-age children, no more than one cup or one can, two or three days weekly.*
- *Preschool children should have no more than half a cup (four ounces) or half a can (six ounces), two or three days weekly.*

For children and teens, emphasize drinking water, low-fat milk, or juice for the majority of meals and snacks. *Strongly discourage* replacing milk with sweetened beverages, such as soft drinks and energy drinks, especially by older children and teens. In addition, be careful regarding energy drinks because they can contain an undesirably high caffeine content. Check product labels. As a point of reference, caffeine in popular soft drinks ranges from 30 to 60 mg.

Stand firm regarding the recommendations for high-calorie foods and sweetened beverages. For those who drink high-calorie beverages, such as soft drinks, be careful not to increase your food intake, especially high-calorie foods. One Sunday, my family and I went to a buffet-type restaurant for lunch. I noticed a customer selecting a Diet Coke. For dessert, she selected a piece of chocolate cream pie. Unfortunately, the Diet Coke does not "cancel" the large number of calories in the chocolate cream pie.

Reducing Eating in Rooms Other Than the Kitchen and Dining Room While Doing Other Activities

Problem

This practice is notorious for promoting overeating.

Recommendations

The ideal way to control such overeating is to eat all meals and snacks in the kitchen or dining area without participating in any other activity. Realistically, however, adults and children enjoy eating a meal or snack in a recreation or family room while watching TV, working on the computer, or reading. If you or other family members give way to such temptation occasionally, that is all right, but keep it to a minimum—it could lead to overeating.

Instead of grabbing a bag of chips or package of cookies, select lighter and more nutritious meals and snacks. For snacks, use a small plate or bowl, custard cup, eight-ounce empty margarine tub, or a small baggie for taco or potato chips (preferably low-fat or whole-grain) or popcorn.

Set a family rule that while doing other activities, you will eat only one meal or snack two or three days weekly in rooms other than the kitchen or dining area. Such a practice helps cut calories and prevents overeating while your attention is focused elsewhere.

Decreasing Meals and Snacks Taken in Fast-Food Establishments or Restaurants

Problem

Many popular selections at restaurants are high in calories, total fat, saturated fat, cholesterol, and sodium. Be sure to check at your local eateries and online products for the levels of such dietary constituents.

Recommendations

To prevent eating excessive amounts of calories and fats, the following tips are recommended when dining out. Select the smart way.

- Look for lighter or portion-controlled meals, often indicated on a menu as "heart healthy," "lighter fare," or "mini-meals."
- Request that bread, rolls, or tortilla-chip baskets be served with the meal instead of before the meal.
- Ask for the lower-fat dressings with your salad, and ask for them to be placed on the side in a separate container.
- Avoid or select only a few items from the appetizer platter, as these are often deep-fat-fried or have a high-fat content.
- Select vegetable soups or broth instead of creamed soups.
- Choose baked, roasted, or grilled meats and fish instead of fried.
- Avoid dishes served with heavy gravies, specialty sauces, cheese, or creamed sauces.
- Opt for a baked potato rather than mashed with gravy, french fries, hash browns, or potato chips.
- Select green beans, carrots, or other green vegetables instead of corn, peas, lima beans, baked beans, or other starchy vegetables.
- Choose toast or bread (preferably whole-grain) or an english muffin, light roll, or bagel instead of a specialty bread (such as banana bread) or a muffin, biscuit, crepe, croissant, or any type of pastry.
- Request a low-fat milk, diet soft drink, water, juice, coffee, or tea instead of a regular soft drink, milkshake, high-calorie coffee beverage, alcoholic beverage, or any type of sweetened beverage.
- Pass on desserts—most of them are high in fat and sugar. Wait until you get home and have some low-fat frozen yogurt, low-fat ice cream, or fruit.
- For sandwiches, opt for roasted or grilled chicken, turkey, fish, or lean beef in lieu of fried meats, bacon, or luncheon meats (such as bologna or salami), which tend to be high in fat.

- Top off your sandwiches with mustard, ketchup, pickles, lettuce, tomatoes, bean sprouts, or other vegetables, rather than mayonnaise, specialty sauces, tartar sauces, or butter or margarine, unless they are a lower-fat variety.
- Order tacos with lettuce and tomato but avoid sour cream and guacamole.
- Try to avoid larger or supersize portions. At an unfamiliar place, if your portion is larger than you expected, share part with a companion or take part of it home to eat later.
- At buffet-type restaurants, remember to take appropriate serving portions; take second helpings only if you really feel hungry. If temptation overcomes you, take a smaller portion of a salad, vegetable, or fruit.
- Beware of children's meals; they often include deep-fat-fried foods such as chicken fingers and french fries.

Be a good example! Though it may be difficult, encourage your children to follow the above recommendations. At the very least, encourage them to take small portions if they choose a selection that's less healthy. All the above recommendations for selecting healthier choices can be applied to eating meals and snacks at home.

You and your family members should eat no more than two days a week at restaurants and fast-food establishments. This applies to take-outs and deliveries as well. Why? In addition to the nutritional reasons given above, this recommendation is based upon the medical findings in *Thorax: An International Journal of Respiratory Medicine* (January 2013). Researcher Phillippa Ellwood and others reported that an increased risk of severe asthma and eczema in teens and children was related to the consumption of fast foods, when eaten three or more days weekly.[2]

Reducing Emotional Overeating

Problem

Emotional overeating can be triggered by stress, boredom, and strong emotions such as anger, frustration, or depression.

Recommendations

By becoming aware of these problematic times, you can be on guard against them. However, in situations when you are stressed or emotionally upset, you may overeat without thinking.

To prevent overeating at these times, "Your Energy Gauge," which should be posted on your refrigerator or cabinet door, can serve to remind you not to open the door. Pause for several minutes to study the different levels of hunger and being full on this gauge and focus on your internal feelings. Ask yourself, "Am I really hungry, or do I want to eat because of boredom, feeling stressed, or because I'm emotionally upset?"

If you do feel hungry, decide at what level and eat according to the dietary recommendations given on the gauge. If you discover that you are not hungry, don't hesitate to take constructive action.

The best strategies to prevent overeating include becoming engaged in physical activity or in a constructive activity that may better appeal to you at the time (e.g., doing crafts, reading a novel). These activities can replace boredom or dispel the destructive physical and mental reactions caused by stress or strong emotions.

It will take practice and patience for you to distinguish your physical feelings of hunger and being full from the psychological need to eat caused by boredom, stress, strong emotions, or by environmental forces, such as social pressure or advertisements.

Children and teens also experience boredom, stress, and strong emotions. Those who are overweight or obese are often teased about their weight or shunned by classmates. Become watchful! If you notice any change in behavior in your child, such as constant eating or becoming withdrawn, ask what is wrong and listen. Assure your child that you love him or her, regardless of his or her weight. By example and instruction, help your child follow the above recommendations. Post lists of physical activities and/or constructive activities for each family member next to "Your Energy Gauge."

Over time, strongly encourage all family members to avoid emotional overeating.

The Importance of Praise and Attention

Giving praise and attention to your children can be powerful rewards. Frequent praise can provide immediate encouragement in a child's or teen's efforts to acquire healthy eating and activity practices. Frequent praise can reinforce the positive changes already made.

Such praise should be specific; for example, "I am proud that you ate your salad." Showing interest in a child's or teen's progress can encourage change.

Endnotes

1   L. L. Birch and J. O. Fisher, "Development of eating behaviors among children and adolescents," *Pediatrics* 101 (1998): 539–549.

2   P. Ellwood et al., "Do fast foods cause asthma, rhinoconjunctivitis and eczema?" *Thorax: A International Journal of Respiratory Medicine* (Jan. 2013).

Chapter 6

Parenting and Promoting Healthy Physical Activity Practices

The focus of the previous chapter was on "calories in"; now let's consider "calories out." Modern conveniences and electronics have contributed to the positive energy state (being overweight or obese) by creating a sedentary lifestyle across the nation that reduces the number of calories expended. Examples of present-day sedentary activities include the following:

- automatic reliance on the family's automobile(s)
- the addictive appeal and use of televisions and computers
- lengthy chatting or texting on cell phones

The recommendations in this chapter will encourage children and teens to become more physically active, while discouraging time spent being inactive. Establishing healthy eating and activity practices will bring the energy equation back into balance so that calories in are equal to calories out. Doing so will reduce the extra calories that have produced unhealthy weight among America's youth.

Becoming Physically Fit as a Family

Physically invest in a healthier future for your family by planning family-centered activities. If you are active, your children will be active too. Join together for such activities as the following:

- brisk walking
- biking
- hiking
- swimming
- skating (ice and roller)
- skiing
- bowling

Other activities could include doing yard work together or cleaning out the garage or basement. Assign specific tasks for each family member, and exchange them from time to time. Have family members plan a family-centered activity once or twice monthly or as often as possible.

Visit the website Shape Up America! (www.shapeupamerica.org). Click on "Children" on the top menu bar, and then click on "Tips for Family Fitness Fun" in the drop-down menu for practical advice on how to personalize family activities. A few of these tips include the following:

- Take turns selecting the activity.
- Select gifts, such as toys or equipment, that promote physical activity.
- Prepare your own nourishing snacks, and have water available at all times.

Most important, emphasize fun and learning over the need to compete. Plan activities with relatives, friends, and neighbors:

- a treasure hunt
- a dancing get-together
- a visit to a farm to pick favorite fruit
- a block fitness festival

Shape Up America! has more specific ideas concerning family-oriented activities.

Parents and their children enjoying a family-centered activity

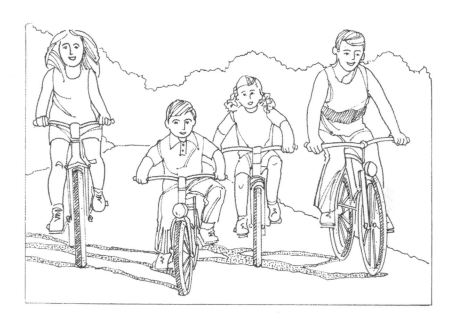

Encouraging Physical Fitness in Your Children: Guidelines to Follow

In the 2015 Dietary Guidelines for Americans, a key recommendation is that children engage in sixty minutes of physical activity daily. Such activities include unstructured play, recreational activities, household and yard chores, sports, and activities promoted by physical education classes. In addition, include stretching and strengthening activities on two or three days of the week for at least twenty minutes each.

Remember to allow a maximum of two hours daily for television and computer viewing. Children under two years of age should not watch television or use computer tablets. The United States Department of Agriculture (www.usda.gov/kidsactivitypyramid) recommends that sedentary activities (or times of inactivity), such as chatting or texting on cell phones, be no more than a half hour daily.

It is important to share with your children and teens the following benefits of the three types of physical activities:[1]

- endurance (including moderate intensity) for a healthy heart
- stretching for flexible joints and muscles
- strengthening for strong muscles and bones

Moderate-intensity activities can include brisk walking, running, biking, swimming, or jumping rope. Such activities raise the heart rate. Have your child place a hand over his or her heart before and after each activity to feel the increase.[2]

Stretching activities could include dancing with stretching arm and leg movements; doing jumping jacks, toe touching (hands over head, reaching to touch toes), or somersaults; and such sports as basketball, baseball, or volleyball.

Strengthening exercises involve weight bearing and could include push-ups, pull-ups, or sit-ups; playing hopscotch; or doing cartwheels.

Take into consideration a child's or teen's age, ability, and interests to increase his or her self-confidence and the likelihood that the child will continue with the activities. This also applies to family-centered activities. Remember to encourage activity early in your child's life.

A Physical Activity Plan for Your Family

Consider the following four-step physical activity plan:

1. Every two weeks, increase moderate-intensity activity by fifteen minutes daily until sixty minutes daily is achieved.
2. Every two weeks, increase strengthening and stretching activities by five minutes each until twenty minutes for each is achieved. These activities should be done on two or three days weekly; choose different days of the week for each activity.
3. Every two weeks, reduce the time spent at the TV or computer for entertainment, starting with four hours, by thirty minutes daily until no more than two hours daily is achieved.

4. Every two weeks, reduce the time spent being inactive (such as chatting or texting on phone), starting with two hours, by thirty minutes daily until no more than a half hour daily is achieved.

If your child or teen spends more time than the starting hours than those given in steps 3 and 4, use the number of hours that are specific to your child or teen as the starting times.

For steps 1 and 2, suggested options include doing one physical activity that day; two activities that day, dividing the time between the two; or doing the activity in shorter episodes, such as four fifteen-minute, three twenty-minute, or two thirty-minute episodes daily. Contact your child's physician to determine if there is an activity that should not be done.

These recommendations apply to parents as well.

An example of a weekly form to keep track of progress is suggested in the following "Building Physical Activity into My Life." After you've duplicated a blank version of this form, have your child write in the moderate-intensity activity or activities that he or she will do that week. After the activities are performed, your child should write in the number of minutes spent on the activities (fifteen, thirty, forty-five, or sixty minutes). The child or teen should then place a gold star or an X (indicating "go") next to the moderate-intensity activities he or she did that day. Next, he or she should write in the strengthening and stretching activities to be done that week and the number of minutes to be spent on those activities (five, ten, fifteen, or twenty minutes). Place a gold star or an X by the stretching or strengthening activity he or she did that day.

Next, add the following two goals: TV and recreational computer time, under two hours, and sitting no more than half an hour. Write in the time spent at the TV/computer (from four to two hours in half-hour increments) and the time spent being inactive (two hours to a half hour, in half-hour increments) for that week. Place a red star or an X (indicating "stop"—inactivity) by each goal if it is met that day. Have your children post this tracking record on the refrigerator or bulletin board for easy access.

If your child or teen engages in the three activities and two additional activities for a week, reinforce his or her efforts with praise. If such practices are met for four weeks, reward him or her. Ideas for rewards can be found in chapter 10, "Promoting Family Responsibility and Health." Remember you may need to begin each activity or goal in small steps and gradually increase or reduce the activity or goal by the number of minutes. This can build self-confidence and increase the likelihood of the activities being continued.

Building Physical Activity into My Daily Routine

- Date to begin: August 1, 2015, and date to end: August 7, 2015. Keep this weekly form to compare to future ones.

• Activity	Minutes	Monday	Tuesday	Wednesday	Thursday	Friday	Saturday	Sunday
Walking	60	x	x	x	x	x	x	x
Push- and Sit-ups	20		x		x			
Dancing	20	x		x				
Limited TV	2 hrs.	x	x	x	x	x	x	x
Inactivity	½ hr.	x	x	x	x	x	x	

Endnotes

1   Canadian Resources, *Canada's Physical Activity Guide to Healthy Active Living: Canada's Physical Activity Guide for Youth* (Kanata, Ontario, Canada: Gilmore, Inc).

2   Canadian Resources, *Canada's Physical Activity Guide to Healthy Active Living: Gotta Move! Magazine for Children 6–9 Years of Age* (Kanata, Ontario, Canada: Gilmore, Inc).

Chapter 7

Promoting a Healthy Weight in Infants and Toddlers

Dr. Elizabeth Jones emphasizes, "A chubby baby is not a healthy baby." Parents need to put into practice the wise words of Benjamin Franklin—"An ounce of prevention is worth a pound of cure"—by keeping pediatric visits for their infants and toddlers. The *most effective* way to confront obesity is to correct the weight problem when it is first identified.

Start with a Healthy Pregnancy

A growing concern in the medical community is that overweight and obese pregnant women have medical problems before and after giving birth. Their infants have a higher risk of physical abnormalities (such as heart and neural tube defects) and developmental disabilities. Physicians recommend that these women reduce their weights as much as possible, preferably within the normal range, before starting a family. It is to the benefit of the infant's and mother's weights that a pregnant woman, regardless of her starting weight, not exceed recommended weight-gain guidelines. In addition, she should follow her doctor's advice regarding recommended dietary intake and activity. The recommendations to promote healthy eating practices in chapter 4 can help to control calories as well.

Weight reduction is not recommended during pregnancy. As a nutrition counselor, one of my responsibilities was to advise expectant mothers on eating a healthy diet and sticking to the weight-gain recommendations. More often than not, the expectant mothers gained more weight than was recommended. I discovered that some of these mothers-to-be were following the age-old but misleading notion that they were "eating for two."

Times of Rapid Growth

Infancy and adolescence are critical periods when obesity could become a problem. Why? The number of calories consumed can influence two biological processes: (1) increase in cell size, and (2) increase in cell number via cellular division. Although other body cells can be affected, the focus here will be on fat cells. When we eat too many calories, fat is deposited, enlarging fat cells, and the number of fat cells are increased. When we eat too few calories, fat is withdrawn, shrinking the fat cells. The number of fat cells, however, *cannot* be reduced. The *higher* the number of fat cells, the *greater* the risk for obesity.

Although not to the same extent, there is another time, around six years of age, when there is a rapid increase in body fat. This is referred to as *adiposity rebound*.[1] Because this rebound could occur even earlier, be alert to your child's increasing his or her dietary intake and weight around this time.[1]

What should parents do? Start by avoiding overfeeding your infants and toddlers. For children and teens, prevent overeating, especially of high-calorie foods and beverages, by following the recommendations given in chapters 1 to 6.

Normal Growth in the Early Years of Life

In the first year of life, there is a rapid rate of growth. For the most part, infants double their birth weight between four and six months of age and triple it by one year. After this first year of rapid growth, the growth rate declines and, at the same time, children's appetites decrease as well.

Because of this, some toddlers and preschoolers become picky eaters, where they limit the number, amount, and type of foods and beverages they eat. For this feeding concern, follow the recommendations given for how to introduce a variety of foods in chapter 1. If such concerns continue, more frequent monitoring of growth and dietary intake may be necessary.

If your child continues to be a picky eater, which may limit his or her intake of nutrients, ask your child's doctor about giving a vitamin and mineral supplement.

Additional information regarding feeding concerns available at www.usda.gov. Type "picky eaters" into the search bar on the top of the screen. This website describes the types of picky eaters and offers suggested steps to take.

Evaluating the Growth of Infants and Toddlers

It is very important to keep pediatric visits. At the initial pediatric visit, the pediatrician will ask questions about your family and medical history and the dietary intake of your infant or toddler. He or she will perform a physical examination on your child and take growth measurements, which will be plotted on the Centers for Disease Control's standard growth charts.

What are these growth charts and what can they tell you about the growth of your infant or toddler?[2]

- These charts include "weight for length, weight for age, length for age, and   head circumference for age".
- Each chart contains percentile curves: "5th, 10th, 25th, 50th, 75th, 90th, and the 95th percentile".
- Let's say, for example, your infant is at the 50th percentile for weight for age. This means that 50 percent of infants weigh less and 50 percent weigh more than your infant at that age.
- As an example of using the weight-for-length growth chart, a mother brought her baby son—a big boy—for a pediatric visit. His weight for his age was at the 90th percentile and his length was at the 90th as well. When his weight was plotted against his length, however, on the weight-for-length growth chart, the weight for length hit around the 50th percentile for age. Why? His weight was balanced by his length.
- As your infant or toddler grows, he or she should track along the initial percentile or between percentiles determined for each chart.

- A measurement below the 5th or above the 95th for any of the growth measurements could indicate a problem that needs to be evaluated.
- Weight for length above the 95th percentile identifies a weight problem. In this case, an infant's weight is too heavy for his or her length.
- It is very important to note when there is any large jump upward across percentile curves on the weight-for-length charts between consecutive visits, especially two or more percentiles, such as from the 25th to the 75th or from the 75th to the 95th.
- An identified weight problem and a large jump upward indicate a medical or overfeeding problem. Your child's physician will determine which of the two problems is contributing to the significant weight gain.
- In the case of a large leap in weight, healthy goals would be to have the weight for length return to the original percentile curve and, in the case of an identified weight problem, return to the normal-weight range; that is, less than the 95th percentile.
- When I evaluated the growth of infants and toddlers at the health department, the standard growth charts were a very important part of the physical examination. I was able to identify not only large leaps in the weight for length, which detected a weight problem, but also large drops, which detected failure to thrive.
- At each doctor visit, ask to see the charts so you can determine where your child's growth parameters place in terms of the percentile curves on each growth chart.
- Ask for a copy of the weight-for-length chart so that charts can be compared, visit by visit. If you have any questions, *do not hesitate* to ask your pediatrician.

I have contacted the CDC numerous times with questions and to request information, and I have always received a prompt reply. I urge you to call the CDC at 800-CDC-Info (800-232-4636) if you have any questions about the growth or weight of your infant or toddler or about other issues; for example, questions about vaccinations.

Steps to Prevent or Correct Excess Weight in Your Infant or Toddler

What can parents do when their child is overweight? It is best that you, as a parent or caregiver, answer the questions below, which will identify the foods and beverages your child eats and drinks that produce extra calories and cause a large leap across weight-for-length percentiles, a current weight problem, or a potential future weight problem. Answer the questions when the child is six, nine, and twelve months of age, and then at eighteen months and two years of age.

Before making any dietary changes, check with your child's physician. Each infant or toddler has unique medical circumstances and family history.

Steps to Take for Your Infant

1. To answer the questions about the different foods and beverages, refer to the following in chapter 2:
   - "Importance of Standard Measurements"
   - "Sample of a Daily Infant Feeding Plan"
   - "High Caloric Foods in the Diets of Infants and Toddlers"

   For each of the foods and beverages listed below ask the following questions, which can identify the problematic foods and beverages that *need to be reduced ("R").*
   - Are you giving a food or beverage *earlier* than the recommended age? If yes, mark as "RE."
   - Are you giving a food or beverage within the basic food groups (dairy to grain), more *often* than recommended in terms of number of times per day? If yes, mark as "RO."
   - Are you giving an infant dessert, combination dinner, or other high-caloric food more *often* than recommended in terms of number of days per week? If yes, mark also as "RO."
   - Are you giving a food or beverage in a larger *amount* than the recommended portion (or serving) size? If yes, mark as "RA."

In some cases, there may be two or three answers. For example, a food may be given too early, too often, and in too large of an amount than recommended—RE RO RA.

2. For the fruit/vegetable and for high-caloric foods, you may wish to write down the particular food or beverage that is causing the problem.

3. Make a list of the following foods and beverages (omit the R's, for they refer to the example):

Dairy Group

    A. Formula *RA*
    B. Milk
    C. Yogurt or Cottage Cheese

Meat/Alternatives Group

    A. Meat or Fish
    B. Cheese
    C. Egg Yolk
    D. Dried Beans or Peas

Fruit/Vegetable Group

    A. Juice *RA*
    B. Other Fruit
    C. Vegetables

Grain Group

    A. Bread
    B. Cereal *RO*
    C. Bun or Bagel
    D. Tortilla
    E. Pasta/Rice
    F. Crackers

Other Foods

    A. Infant Desserts *RE RO*
    B. Infant Combination Dinners with Gravy
    C. Other High-Caloric Foods

4. Adhere to the following dietary recommendations:
   - If a food or beverage is marked as RE (too early), reduce the food or beverage over one to two weeks until no longer given, and reintroduce it at the appropriate age.
   - If a food or beverage is marked as RE (too early) and RO (too often), reduce the food or beverage over one to two weeks until no longer given, and reintroduce it at the appropriate age and at the recommended number of times daily or days weekly.
   - If a food or beverage is marked as RE (too early) and RA (too large of an amount), reduce the food or beverage over one to two weeks until no longer given, and reintroduce it at the appropriate age and at the recommended amount.
   - If a food or beverage is marked as RE (too early), RO (too often), and RA (too large of an amount), reduce the food or beverage over two to three weeks until no longer given, and reintroduce it at the appropriate age and at the recommended amount and recommended times daily or days weekly.
   - If a food or beverage is marked as RO (too often) or RA (too large of an amount), reduce the food or beverage over one to two weeks until the recommended amount or recommended number of times daily or days weekly is reached.
   - If a food or beverage is marked as RO (too often) and RA (too large of an amount), reduce the food or beverage over two to three weeks until the recommended amount and recommended number of times daily or days weekly are reached.
   - High-caloric (sweetened) beverages are not recommended for infants. If you are giving such a beverage, reduce

it over one to two weeks until no longer given and reintroduce it at the appropriate age.

- To determine the total number of weeks that it takes to reduce all the problematic foods and beverages, add up the individual weeks required for each of the foods and beverages.

Here is an example set of dietary recommendations for an infant:

- A mother is giving her infant a fruit-type dessert at six months (RE) and on three days of the week (RO). She needs to reduce this dessert over one to two weeks and then reintroduce it at eight months at the recommended one or two days weekly.
- She is giving 40 ounces of formula daily. She needs to reduce this formula over one to two weeks until the recommended 24 to 32 ounces is reached.
- She is giving two ounces of undiluted juice (RA). She needs to reduce this beverage over one to two weeks until the recommended one ounce diluted, daily, is reached.
- She is giving one to two tablespoons of cereal three times daily (RO). She needs to reduce this food over one to two weeks until the food is given only twice daily.
- The total number of weeks to make all reductions is four to eight weeks.

5. Return to the list of foods and beverages to see how the problem foods and beverage are identified by the specific abbreviations.
6. After each month, until all reductions are made, check with his or her physician. He or she may wish to do a weight check to reevaluate weight status and, if needed, further advise.
   - Keep a record of weights.
   - If there are extra calories and a weight gain that is above that required for normal growth, these steps will remove the extra calories in order to prevent additional weight gain.

- *If the problem is a large leap across weight-for-length percentiles, the goal is to have the weight for length return to the initial percentile for age.*
- *If there is a weight problem, the goal is to have the weight for length fall below the 95th percentile for age.*

Steps to Take for Your Toddler

1. Encourage safe physical activity. If you have questions, ask his or her physician.
2. To answer the questions about the different foods and beverages, refer to the following in chapter 2:
   - "Importance of Standard Measurements"
   - "Recommended Food and Beverage Intakes for Toddlers"
   - "High-Caloric Foods in the Diets of Infants and Toddlers"

   For each of the foods and beverages listed below, ask the following questions, which can identify the problematic foods and beverages that *need to be reduced ("R")*.
   - Are you giving more servings for a food group (dairy to fat) than the recommended *number* of servings daily? If yes, mark as "RN."
   - Are you giving a food or beverage in a larger *amount* than the recommended portion (or serving) size? If yes, mark as "RA."
   - Are you giving a high-caloric food more *often* than recommended in terms of number of days per week? If yes, mark as "RO."

   In some cases, there may be two answers. For example, a food may be given too often and in too large of an amount than recommended—"RO RA."

3. For the fruit/vegetable and high-caloric foods, you may wish to write down the particular food or beverage that is causing the problem.
4. Make a list of the following foods and beverages (omit the R's, for they refer to the example):

Dairy Group

A. Milk
B Yogurt

Meat/Alternatives Group

A. Meat or Fish
B. Cheese
C. Egg
D. Dried Beans or Peas
E. Peanut Butter

Fruit/Vegetable Group

A. Juice
B. Other Fruit *RA Banana*
C. Vegetables

Grain Group *RN*

A. Bread
B. Cereal
C. Bun or Bagel
D. Tortilla
E. Pasta/Rice
F. Crackers

Fat Group

A. Butter
B. Margarine
C. Mayonnaise
D. Salad Dressing
E. Cream Cheese

Other Foods

High-Caloric Foods *RO* Vanilla Wafers

5. Adhere to the following dietary recommendations:
    *   If a food group is marked as RN (more than the number of servings recommended), reduce the number of servings over one to two weeks until the recommended number is reached.
    *   If a food or beverage is marked as RO (too often) or RA (too large of an amount), reduce the food or beverage over one to two weeks until the recommended amount or number of days weekly is reached.
    *   If a food or beverage is marked as RO (too often) and RA (too large of an amount), reduce the food or beverage over two to three weeks until the recommended amount and number of days weekly are reached.
    *   High-caloric (sweetened) beverages are not recommended for toddlers. If you are giving such a beverage, reduce it over one to two weeks until no longer given, and reintroduce it at the appropriate age at recommended levels.
    *   To determine the total number of weeks that it takes to reduce all the problematic foods and beverages, add up the individual weeks required for each of the foods and beverages.

    Here is an example set of dietary recommendations for a toddler:
    *   A toddler is eating eight servings from the grain group (RN). The mother should reduce the number of servings over one to two weeks until the recommended six servings daily is reached.
    *   A toddler is eating one small banana (RA). The mother should reduce the banana over one to two weeks until only a fourth to a half is eaten daily.
    *   A toddler is eating two to three vanilla wafers four days (RO). The mother should reduce the vanilla wafers over

one to two weeks until they are given only one or two days weekly.

- The total amount of time needed to make the recommendations is three to six weeks.

6. Return to the list of foods and beverages to see how the problem foods are identified by the specific abbreviations.
7. After each month, until all reductions are made, check with his or her physician. He or she may wish to do a weight check to reevaluate weight status and, if needed, further advise.
   - Keep a record of weights.
   - If there are extra calories and a weight gain that is above that required for normal growth, these steps will remove the extra calories in order to prevent additional weight gain.
   - *If the problem is a large leap across weight-for-length (or stature) percentiles, the goal is to have the weight for length (or stature) return to the initial percentile for age.*
   - *If there is a weight problem, the goal is to have the weight for length (or stature) fall below the 95th percentile for age.*

Endnotes

1   "Seminars in Nutrition," *Obesity: Assessment, Risks, and Management* 19 (1999): 1–16.
2   Growth Charts, National Center for Health Statistics, Centers for Disease Control. Permission has been given to include information from the Centers for Disease Control with the following disclaimer statements: Links to nonfederal organizations are provided as a service. Links are not an endorsement of these organizations or their programs by CDC or the federal government. CDC is not responsible for the content of organization websites found at these links.
    Thank you for contacting CDC-INFO. For more information, please call 1-800-CDC-INFO (800-232-4636), visit www.cdc.gov and click on "Contact CDC-INFO," or go to www.cdc.gov/info. If you have questions or comments, please send them via our online form at www.cdc.gov/info. CDC-INFO is a service of the Centers for Disease Control and Prevention (CDC) and the Agency for Toxic Substances and Disease Registry (ATSDR). This service is provided by Verizon and its subcontractors under the Networx Universal contract to CDC and ATSDR.

Chapter 8

Promoting a Healthy Weight in Children and Teens

Without a doubt, childhood obesity has become a serious public health concern. At any age, an excessive rate of weight gain relative to growth in height should be recognized[1] so that measures to correct the weight problem can be taken. As previously mentioned, extra weight is responsible for the early presence of serious medical and psychological problems for children and teens; for example, high blood pressure, high blood levels of glucose, and high cholesterol. If not corrected, these complications, like the weight problem that caused them, will continue into adulthood. They will worsen and can trigger such chronic diseases as cardiovascular disease (heart disease, high blood pressure, stroke) and type 2 diabetes. These chronic diseases can lead to compromised health or disability, as well as a shortened life expectancy.

Devastating also are the psychological problems (e.g., poor body image, low self-esteem), emotional problems (e.g., depression, frustration), and social problems (e.g., isolation, embarrassment) experienced by children with weight difficulties. For example, my sister was looking at the corner where children were gathering to wait for their school bus. There were several children interacting, but at a distance stood a boy who was overweight. This was a heart-breaking view. Such medical consequences and psychological scars are the price tags that our children and teens pay for being obese.

Normal Growth in Children and Teens

Except for the risk of adiposity rebound around six years of age, as described in chapter 7, growth settles into a steady rate for school-age children.

During the teen years, there is a rapid rate of growth, referred to as the adolescent growth spurt. There are two nutritional concerns related to this growth spurt. First, male teens gain muscle mass, while teen girls gain body fat. Because of the undesirable weight gain, some teen girls develop an eating disorder. Second, maximum skeletal mineralization takes place at this time. As mentioned in chapter 2, a number of older children and teens are replacing milk with soft drinks and energy drinks. This reduction in calcium can compromise both skeletal growth (height) and skeletal strength.

Evaluating the Growth of Children and Teens

- *It is very important to keep pediatric visits.* For children two years old through teenage, you will be asked questions about his or her dietary and activity practices at each visit. You will need to provide updated information about your family's medical history as well. A physical exam (including a blood pressure reading) will be done. If needed, the physician may order a laboratory work-up for the testing of glucose or cholesterol.
- As with infants and toddlers, your child's or teen's growth measurements will be taken and plotted on standard growth charts.
- These growth charts include "BMI for Age, Weight for Age, and Stature for Age". For example, included here is the BMI For age for boys. see "CDC Growth charts: United States:
- In addition, there is a "85th on the BMI for Age chart".
- Note that the BMI percentiles are determined by the relationship between weight and height.
- As children and teens grow, they should track along the same percentile curves or between curves for each growth parameter.

- BMI percentiles for age determines their weight status. These percentiles for age for children and teens should be plotted yearly.
- Based upon standard growth charts for age and sex, consider children and adolescents with BMI percentiles from the 85th to 94th percentiles as overweight and at or above the 95th percentiles as obese.[1,2]
- Large jumps upward across percentile curves, especially two or more (such as from the 50th to the 85th) between yearly visits could indicate a medical or overeating problem. This also applies to children and teens who have an overweight or obesity problem.
- In the case of a large leap in weight, healthy goals would be to have the BMI for age return to the original percentile curve.
- In the case of an identified weight problem, the goal is to be less than the 85th percentile; For both an overweight or obese problem and for large leaps in weight gain, the physician should be able to determine the problem contributing to the excessive weight gain. Recommendations to correct such weight concerns will be discussed shortly.
- Ask to see where your child's or teen's growth parameters place on the percentile curves on each growth chart.
- Ask for a copy of the BMI-for-age chart and any laboratory results, if done, so that they can be compared, visit by visit.
- Also keep a note of the blood pressure reading and if it was normal or abnormal.
- If you would like to see a more detailed discussion of these standard percentiles, the CDC invites parents to calculate percentiles for children and teens at any time, as well as offering helpful tips on how to correct weight problems.
- Explore www.cdc.gov/bmipercentilecalculatorforchildand teens. I urge you to call the CDC at 800-CDC-Info (800-232-4636) if you have any questions about the growth or weight of your child or teen or about other issues; for example, vaccinations.

CDC Growth Charts: United States

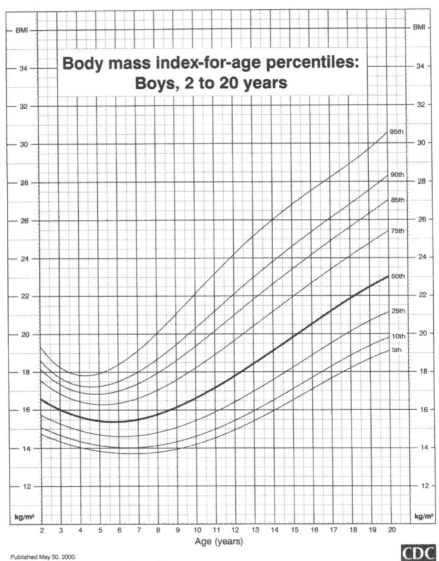

BMI Percentiles for Age for Boys

Recommended Laboratory Testing

Laboratory tests may be recommended by your child's physician and will be based, for example, upon age, medical and family histories of disease, and results from the physical examination. This work-up generally includes testing for glucose, cholesterol (HDL and LDL), and triglyceride levels, which indicate whether the fasting levels are normal or abnormal. Such results are important, as they can help determine which weight control measures to take—either weight maintenance or the amount of weight to lose.

Review the results with the physician, and request a copy of the results so you can compare them with the results of future testing, if treatment is required. Such requests are especially important if there is a strong history of obesity, hypertension, cardiovascular disease, or type 2 diabetes.

Medical Information: What Should Parents Do?

Parents should keep a record of the date of each child's physician visit, as well as the following:

- age
- height and weight
- BMI percentiles for age
- results of the physical examine, blood pressure readings, and laboratory work-ups (Circle abnormal blood pressure readings, weight-related physical findings, and/or laboratory results.)
- any weight-related medical complications caused by abnormal findings
- advice given for diet, physical activity, or referral for each abnormal finding
- date of visit(s) when each abnormal finding was corrected or additional advice given

Important Precautions

Several precautions need to be addressed:

- Certain categories of medications for adults can cause weight gain or interfere with weight loss. If any of these categories of drugs have been prescribed for your child or teen or if you have noticed that a particular drug has produced a weight gain, consult his or her physician for an alternate medication. Additional resources of information could include a local registered pharmacist, registered dietitian, or public health nutritionist, or you could investigate the prescribed medication via the Internet.
- Adult dietary supplements are not recommended for children and teens. Not only are the safety and effectiveness questionable for many supplements, but adult dosages levels are not appropriate for children and teens. Additionally, certain dietary supplements can interfere with the actions of prescribed medications.
- Adult weight-loss programs or popular fad diets are not recommended for children and teens.

Parents with weight problems often have children with weight problems, especially when both parents are overweight or obese. Although genetics may play a part, environmental influences, involving both unhealthy eating and activity practices, are the greater factor in creating weight problems. Because of this, the purpose of the weight-control recommendations presented below for children and teens is to acquire healthy eating and activity practices, which then can promote the desired weight maintenance or loss.

Specific Weight-Management Recommendations for Children and Teens

Your child's or teen's physician will recommend one of the following: (1) weight maintenance, (2) a gradual weight loss of one pound per month, or (3) a one- or two-pound loss per week. The purpose of weight maintenance is to hold your child's or teen's weight constant, while height continues to increase. This allows the relationship between height and weight to reach a normal weight range.

When the physician recommends a gradual weight loss of one pound per month, this is a reduction of one hundred calories from the daily dietary intake. If a more rapid weight loss of one or two pounds per day is recommended, this would represent a decrease of 500–1,000 calories from the daily dietary intake. Because this would be a significant reduction, especially for teens (because of a high nutrient demand for growth), they would require close supervision by a physician or registered dietitian.

The physician's decision regarding the above recommendations will depend upon the following for your child or teen:

1. Age
2. BMI percentile and weight status (normal, overweight, or obese)
3. A family history of obesity and/or weight-related chronic diseases (e.g., heart disease, diabetes, high blood pressure)
4. Abnormal findings identified by blood pressure readings, physical examination, or laboratory results
5. Weight-related medical complications caused by such abnormal findings

Even small positive changes in weight and physical activity can produce significant improvement in weight-related medical complications. These positive changes can encourage parents to continue the eating and activity practices that brought about such results. The changes also can encourage your child or teen for further weight loss, if required. It would be best to continue weight-maintenance or weight-loss recommendations until the medical complication is corrected.

For children or teens with serious weight problems, pediatric obesity specialists recommend the "Weight-control Information Network (WIN)."[3] For these services, which have experience with serious pediatric weight problems, contact WIN at 877-946-4627 or at www.win@info.niddk.nih.gov. You may wish to phone WIN and ask for local hospitals or medical facilities for pediatric weight-related services near you.

Steps to Prevent or Correct Excess Weight in Preschool and School-Age Children and Teens

It is best that you, as a mother or father (or caregiver), answer the questions given below about the foods and beverages that your child or teen is eating.

- These questions can identify the foods and beverages that produce extra calories that are *causing a large leap across BMI percentiles or a current weight problem or that could create one in the future.*
- It is advised here that a parent of a child or teen answer the questions every six months.
- *Before making any dietary changes, check with his or her physician because every child or teen has unique medical circumstances and family histories.*

1. For preschool children, encourage them to enjoy a variety of age-appropriate physical activities. If you have any questions, check with his or her physician.

    For school-age children and teens, increase moderate-intensity physical activities by fifteen minutes daily until the recommended sixty minutes daily is achieved. See "A Physical Activity Plan for Your Family" (chapter 6).
    - For these age groups, you may wish to use the "Building Physical Activity into My Life" (chapter 6) to track progress.
    - Contact his or her physician. There may be a physical activity that should not be done.

2. To answer the questions about the different foods and beverages, refer to
    - "Importance of Standard Measurements" (chapter 2)
    - "Recommended Food and Beverage Intakes for Preschoolers" (chapter 3)
    - "High-Caloric Foods and Beverages in the Diets of Preschoolers" (chapter 3)
    - For school-age children and teens, the "Serving Sizes Recommended by the USDA" and "Dietary Plans for

Children and Teens" appearing after step 9 (Note the dietary plan for your child or teen is based upon age.)
- "High-Calorie Foods and Beverages in the Diets of School-Age Children & Teens (chapter 3)

With the help of your child or teen, write down the intake of your child or teen for three days. Include one weekend and two weekdays that best reflect his or her *typical* intake.
- For each meal and snack, write down the foods and beverages given and the amounts.
- Ask him or her how many days weekly and in what amounts he or she is eating high-caloric foods (cookies, candy, potato chips, etc.).
- Ask him or her how many days weekly and in what amounts he or she is drinking high-caloric beverages (soft or energy drinks, Kool-Aid, etc.).
- Emphasize to him or her that it is important to include all foods and beverages, including the high-caloric ones.
- A set of standard measuring cups can be helpful in aiding your child or teen to learn about the amount of foods and beverages consumed.
- Weekly menus from schools and day care centers can also be helpful.

This will take time and patience, but having a healthy child or teen is worth the effort.

3. For each of the foods and beverages listed below, ask the following questions, which can identify the problematic foods and beverages that *need to be reduced ("R")*.
   - Is your child or teen eating more servings for a food group (dairy to fat) than the recommended *number* of servings daily? If yes, mark as "RN."
   - Is your child or teen eating a food or beverage in a larger *amount* than the recommended portion (or serving) size? If yes, mark as "RA."

- Is your child or teen eating a high-caloric food more *often* than recommended in terms of number of days per week? If yes, mark as "RO."
- Is your child or teen drinking a high-caloric beverage more *often* than recommended in terms of number of days per week? If yes, mark as "RO."

In some cases, there may be two answers. For example, a food may be given too often and in too large of an amount than recommended—RO RA.

4. Some children and teens are replacing milk with soft drinks and energy beverages. At the same time, they are replacing fruits and vegetables with high-caloric foods. Because of these replacements, ask the questions below in order *to increase* "I," the consumption of milk and fruits and vegetables.
    - Is your child eating less than the *number* of servings of dairy products than is recommended daily? If yes, mark as "IN."
    - Is your child eating a smaller *amount* of a dairy product than the recommended portion (or serving size daily)? If yes, mark as "IA."
    - Is your child eating less than the *number* of servings of fruits and vegetables than the recommended number of servings daily? If yes, mark as "IN."
    - Is your child eating a smaller *amount* of a fruit or vegetable than the recommended portion (or serving size daily)? If yes, mark as "IA."

5. For the fruit/vegetable and high-caloric foods and beverages, you may wish to write down the particular food or beverage that is causing the problem.
6. Make a list of the following foods and beverages (omit the R's and I's, for they refer to the example):

Dairy Group *IN*

    A. Milk
    B Yogurt

Meat/Alternatives Group

A. Meat or Fish
B. Cheese
C. Egg
D. Dried Beans or Peas
E. Peanut Butter

Fruit/Vegetable Group *IN*

A. Juice
B. Other Fruit
C. Vegetables

Grain Group

A. Bread
B. Cereal
C. Bun or Bagel
D. Tortilla
E. Pasta/Rice
F. Crackers

Fat Group

A. Butter
B. Margarine
C. Mayonnaise
D. Salad Dressing
E. Cream Cheese

Other Foods

A. High-Caloric Foods *RO Candy Bar*
B. High-Caloric Beverages *RO Soft Drink*

7. Adhere to the following dietary recommendations:
   - If a food group is marked as RN (more than the number of servings recommended), reduce the number of servings over one to two weeks until the recommended number is reached.
   - If a food or beverage is marked as RO (too often) or RA (too large of an amount), reduce the food or beverage over one to two weeks until the recommended amount or number of days weekly is reached.
   - If a food or beverage is marked as RO (too often) and RA (too large of an amount), reduce the food or beverage over two to three weeks until the recommended amount and number of days weekly are reached.
   - If a food or beverage is marked as IN, increase the food or beverage over one to two weeks until the recommended number of servings daily is reached.
   - If a food or beverage is marked as IA, increase the food or beverage over one to two weeks until the recommended amount daily is achieved.
   - To determine the total number of weeks that it takes to reduce all the problematic foods and beverages, add up the individual weeks required for each of the foods and beverages.

Here is an example set of dietary recommendations for a ten-year-old child:
   - Your child is eating a candy bar daily (RO). Have him or her reduce this over one to two weeks until the recommended three or four days weekly is reached.
   - Your child is drinking a can of soft drink every day (RO). Have him or her reduce this over one to two weeks until the recommended two or three days weekly is reached.
   - Your child is eating only two servings of fruit and vegetables (IN). Have him or her increase the number of servings over one to two weeks until the recommended five servings daily is reached.
   - Your child is eating one serving of a dairy product daily (IN). Have him or her increase the number of servings

over one to two weeks until the recommended three servings daily is reached.

- The total time needed for all reductions and increases is four to eight weeks.

8. Return to the list of foods and beverages to see how the problem foods and beverages are identified by the specific abbreviations.

9. After each month, until all reductions and increases are made, check with his or her physician. He or she may wish to do a weight check to reevaluate weight status and, if needed, further advise.

- Keep a record of weights.
- If there are extra calories and a weight gain that is above that required for normal growth, these steps will remove the extra calories in order to prevent additional weight gain.
- If the problem is a large leap across BMI percentiles, the goal is to have the BMI return to the initial percentile for age.
- If the problem is an overweight or obese status, the goal is to have the BMI fall below the 85th percentile for age.

Serving Sizes Recommended by the USDA

Dairy Products

- One serving is 8 ounces (1 cup) of milk or 6–8 ounces (3/4–1 cup) of yogurt.
- It is best to select fat-free or low-fat (1 percent) products.
- If 2 percent milk is preferred, count as two servings of milk *plus* one serving of fat in the dietary plan.

Meat and Meat Alternatives

For meats, determine amount after cooking and after removing bones, skin, and fat from the edges of meat. A 4-ounce piece of raw meat will yield 3 ounces of cooked meat.

As often as possible, select lean cuts of meat, lean hamburger, and low-fat luncheon meats, hot dogs, cheese, and peanut butter.

An average portion of meat and an alternative is 2 or 3 ounces. This could include 2 or 3 ounces of poultry, meat, or fish; 2 or 3 ounces of sandwich meats; 2 ounces (1/4 cup) of tuna (water-packed or drained of oil); or 2 or 3 ounces of cheese. An ounce of meat or an alternative can include 1 hot dog, 1 egg, 1 tablespoon of peanut butter, or 1/2 cup of dried beans or peas.

Consider the dimensions of four inches by three inches and a half-inch thick as 3 ounces of a patty, set of thin slices, or a piece of meat. Examples include half a chicken breast; a regular-sized hamburger, tenderloin, or pork chop; or chicken or fish fillet. In addition, consider a wing of chicken to be 1 ounce and the leg and thigh as 2 ounces.

- Two ounces of cheese is two thin slices or the size of a two-inch square chunk.
- Meat and alternatives with a higher fat content can be consumed. Count as one serving of the following plus one serving of fat in the dietary plan:

1. Each ounce of prime cuts
2. Each ounce of other meats high in fat (e.g., meatloaf, ground beef, bacon)
3. Each ounce of sandwich meats (bologna, pastrami) and 1 hot dog
4. Each ounce of American, Swiss, cheddar, jack, mozzarella or other cheeses
5. Each ounce of fried chicken or fish
6. Each egg, scrambled or fried
7. Each tablespoons of peanut butter

Because of the high fat content, whether one, two, or three ounces or tablespoons, consume only one or two of such foods, no more than once or twice weekly.

Fruits and Vegetables

> 4 ounces juice
> 1 small piece of fruit
> 1/2 cup berries or other fruits
> 1 cup melon
> 1/4 cup dried fruits

One serving of vegetables is any one of the following:

> 1/2 cup cooked vegetables
> 1/2 cup chopped raw vegetables or sticks
> 1 cup leafy raw vegetables (lettuce or spinach)
> 3/4 cup vegetable juice

Quite often, children and teens prefer corn and potatoes, especially french fries, which have a higher fat content. For each small serving or package of french fries, count as one serving of vegetable *plus* one serving of fat in the dietary plan. Corn and potatoes and other vegetables such as peas and lima beans contain a higher content of carbohydrates. Because of this, it is best to offer these vegetables at a meal only on three or four days weekly.

You may wish to offer a colorful vegetable plus a serving of a whole-grain pasta or wild rice.

Breads, Cereals, and Pastas (Grains)

One serving (preferably whole-grain) is any one of the following:

> a slice of bread or small roll
> 1/2 hamburger or hot dog bun
> 1/2 small bagel (1 ounce) or 1/2 english muffin
> 6 small or 3 to 4 large crackers
> 1/2 cup cooked cereal, rice, or pasta
> 3/4 cup (1 ounce) of ready-to-eat cereal (lower
> added sugar preferred)
> A small biscuit or muffin can be eaten occasionally.

Fats and Oils

One serving is any one of the following:

> 1 teaspoon margarine, butter, mayonnaise, or vegetable oil
> 1 tablespoons salad dressing, cream cheese, or sour cream
> Select fat-free, low-fat, reduced-fat, or light products.

Other Foods and Beverages

Some foods and beverages contain very few calories; that is, less than twenty-five calories per servings. Such foods and beverages can be included into the dietary intake without considering them in the total daily intake of calories. These include condiments, such as mustard and ketchup; coffee, tea, and diet soft drinks; and certain fat-free products. Check product labels for calories per serving and serving size.

Dietary Plans for Children and Teens

Note: The numbers given under the food groups represent "number of servings," except for the Meat and Meat Alternatives group, which represent "ounces." The third serving of a calcium-rich source for children 9 to 12 years and teens could be 2 ounces of cheese, which, for the purposes of these dietary plans, is included under the Meat and Meat Alternatives group.

Meat and alternatives are given as Meat/Alt, vegetables as Veg, and extra calories as EX. Extra calories can be used for commercial products, preferably nourishing ones. Check the product label for serving size and calories per serving. Age is in years.

Age	Dairy	Meat/Alt	Fruit	Veg	Grain	Fat	Extra
Girls							
5–8	2	5	3	2	6	2	0
9–10	2	6	3	2	7	3	0
11–13	2	7	4	2	8	3	0
14–18	2	7	4	3	10	4	0
Boys							
5–8	2	6	3	2	7	3	0
9–10	2	7	4	2	8	3	0
11–12	2	7	4	3	10	4	0
13–14	2	8	4	3	11	5	0
15–18	2	8	4	3	11	5	200

Example of a Dietary Plan

For an example of a dietary plan see the "Dietary Plan for Girls Five to Eight Years" on the following pages. This plan has three meals and two snacks. If the typical eating pattern of your child or teen has more snacks, use food groups assigned to the three meals for these snacks. For other dietary plans for both boys and girls, you can add the necessary number of food groups (and extra calories, if available) to this dietary plan until they match the number of food groups given for the specific recommended dietary plan for your child or teen.

The foods and beverages given on the plan are only examples. Refer to the "Serving Sizes Recommended by the USDA" for other food and beverage options.

Dietary Plan for Girls Five to Eight Years

Recommended number of food groups

- 2 servings dairy
- 5 servings meat/alternatives
- 3 servings fruit
- 2 servings vegetables
- 6 servings grain
- 2 servings fat
- 0 servings extra calories

Breakfast Sample Menu

1 grain	3/4 cup unsweetened cereal, bagel (1 ounce), or 1 slice toast
1 milk	1 cup 1 percent milk or 6 ounces fat-free yogurt
1 fruit	1/2 cup orange juice, small banana, or medium peach
1 fat	1 teaspoon soft margarine or 1/2 tablespoon peanut butter
other	2 teaspoons light jam, 1 tablespoons fat-free cream cheese, or 1 teaspoons reduced-fat margarine

Lunch

2 grain	2 slices bread, 1 bun, or bagel (2 ounces)
2 meat	2 ounces sandwich meat, 2 ounces cheese, or 2 tablespoons of peanut butter
1 vegetable	1 cup carrot sticks, celery, or broccoli (raw)
1 fruit	1/2 cup apple juice, 1 small orange, or 1/2 cup pears
1 fat	1 teaspoon soft margarine or 2 tablespoons reduced-fat Miracle Whip

Dinner

1 grain	1 slice bread, 1 small roll, or bagel (1 ounce)
3 meat	3 ounces chicken, beef, pork, or fish
1 vegetable	1/2 cup green beans, spinach, etc.
1 vegetable	1 cup tomato wedges
1 fat	1 teaspoons soft margarine or 2 tablespoons reduced-fat salad dressing
1 milk	1 cup 1 percent milk or 6 ounces fat-free yogurt
other	2 slices bread-and-butter pickles or lettuce

Snack (s)

1 grain	3 graham crackers (2 half-inch squares), 8 animal crackers, or 4 whole-wheat crackers
1 fruit	1 small apple, 1 cup cantaloupe, or 1 1/4 cup strawberries
other	2 tablespoons light whipped topping

Practical Pointers to Help You Keep a Handle on Your Teen's Dietary Intake

Consider the following suggestions to reduce your teen's reliance on fast food and beverages:

1. Remember to acquire a weekly meal schedule from his or her school so that you can coordinate meals and snacks between home and school.
2. Have your teen prepare healthy lunches.

3. Limit the money he or she takes to school to decrease the purchase of high-calorie foods and beverages.

Teens' dietary patterns are characterized by the following:

- Hectic eating with meals skipped
- Many meals and snacks consumed outside of the home, where popular purchases are less nourishing and eaten in larger portion sizes
- Fewer meals and more snacks consumed

Weight management for many teens can be challenging, but persuade the teen with a weight problem to consider the recommendations presented below.

First, have your teen establish a less hectic schedule. Help him or her to plan a healthy schedule of activities (see chapter 4).

Second, have your teen take the following steps related to dietary intake (the first five recommendations also can be applied to eleven- to twelve-year-olds):

1. Explore the websites for the fast-food establishments where favorite foods and beverages are purchased. Then, write down the number of calories for each item.
2. For foods and beverages purchased at school snack bars, concession stands, school stores, à la carte options, or vending machines, search for fast-food products to acquire calorie values that can be assigned to similar school-related selections. Then, write down the popular school-related products and the assigned calorie values.
3. Next, from these sites select healthier alternatives that are lower in calories, fat, sugar, and sodium to replace both the fast food and school-related foods and beverages, and write down their calorie values.
4. Keep a two- or three-week log of the fast food and school-related products, including the date, day, time, place, the specific food and beverage purchased, the amount and number of calories of each item, and a total number of calories contributed by these purchases for each week.

By doing this log, teens can realize the large number of calories that can be consumed by these unhealthy products; the specific foods and beverages that are especially high in calories and consumed frequently; and when and where such calorie-costly items can be replaced by healthier ones.

5. Have him or her keep a list of favorite fast-food products and the healthier alternatives and the number of calories for each.

6. No more than four hundred calories from fast-food-type products purchased in the community or at school should be consumed for a dietary plan for girls ages eleven to thirteen years and for boys ages eleven and twelve years; no more than six hundred for dietary plans for girls ages fourteen to eighteen years and boys thirteen and fourteen years; and no more than eight hundred calories for dietary plans for boys ages fifteen to eighteen years. To meet such calorie limitations, encourage your teen to opt for healthier alternatives and avoid supersize or jumbo selections.

7. The dietary plans for girls and boys are separated by approximately two hundred calories. To keep the daily total calorie intake similar, an example is given here. A boy, fourteen years old, consuming six hundred calories from fast-food-type products, should follow the dietary plan for boys five to eight years for foods and beverages consumed in the home.

Third, have your teen become as physically active as possible. See "A Physical Activity Plan for Your Family" (chapter 6).

In addition, share his or her dietary plan with your teen and the recommendations for meals and snacks for teens in chapter 4. Your teen *must* realize the importance of acquiring a healthy weight and act upon this belief.

Helping Your Children Become Psychologically Fit

Media and social messages promote the idea that being super-thin is required to be attractive, popular, and successful. As a result, an unhealthy focus upon weight and dissatisfaction with their bodies occurs, especially among girls. This can trigger unhealthy eating practices.

It is important to be watchful of the dietary practices of children and teens, as well as the types of information they are exposed to via printed or Internet information.

Work hard to convince your children, especially teens, that the media's message promoting super-thinness is an unhealthy ideal. Rather, explain there is a healthy weight range for each individual. Emphasize that weight should not be the standard for judging a person's worth or acceptance. How can these healthy beliefs be reinforced by parental actions? To downplay weight as the central focus in the minds of children and teens, do the following actions often:

- Hug and kiss your children, and tell them that you love them, especially those who have a weight problem.
- Compliment your child and teen on his or her beautiful smile, sharing with other children, being friendly, getting good grades, athletic ability, and so on.
- Strongly discourage weight-related criticisms and actions, especially among siblings.
- Assign each child or teen a small task, such as for the household or yard, and gradually add more difficult ones to promote confidence and a positive self-esteem.
- To show your respect for individuals of different sizes and shapes, point out important qualities in relatives and friends, such as caring, willingness to help, or being reliable.
- Periodically reward your children and teens with a smile or praise for positive comments about others, regardless of the person's weight.

Concerning the psychologically based eating disorders, if you practice dietary restraint, yo-yo dieting (repeated cycles of gain and loss), or any other eating disorder, work hard to improve your own eating and activity practices, or seek professional help along with your teen. Do not become an example or impose such unhealthy eating practices on your child or teen, whether or not he or she has a weight problem.

Become alert to whether your child or teen is overly concerned about or dissatisfied with his or her weight, becomes depressed or withdrawn, reduces food intake, or skips meals. In addition, carefully watch your children, especially teens, for signs of starving, binge eating, or vomiting after meals. These disorders are very serious and should be caught early. If you observe such practices, emphasize to your teen that good eating and activity practices can help prevent compromised health during the significant growth taking place in his or her life. If you see any evidence of such unhealthy behaviors being continued, contact his or her physician. Ask his or her physician to refer you to a professional experienced in the area of eating disorders.

Carefully read the following chapter on setting healthy goals for the family; it summarizes the eating and activity recommendations in specific detail, as presented in the previous chapters. Efforts to change unhealthy eating and activity practices will take time, effort, and patience, but they will be worthwhile, as they will ensure a happier and healthier family.

Endnotes

1   S. E. Barlow and W. H. Dietz, "Obesity evaluation and treatment: Expert committee recommendations," *Pediatrics* 120 (2007): S164–S192.
2   Growth Charts, National Center for Health Statistics, Center for Disease Control.
3   S. E. Barlow and W. H. Dietz, "Obesity evaluation and treatment: Expert committee recommendations" *Pediatrics* 102 (1998): 1–11.

Chapter 9

Setting Healthy Goals for the Family

Within my training in public health, it was emphasized that setting goals is *key* to making changes. I strongly recommend that you and your family members set healthy goals that focus on eating and activity practices that need to be improved. In addition, positive changes should be as follows:

- reasonable in terms of being able to achieve and able to continue
- considered as lifelong practices, not quick-fix changes
- establish healthy eating and activity practices in the early years (making such changes in older children and teens is more difficult)

Family Meetings to Set Healthy Goals

Family meetings should be held every three months to determine healthy goals. Family meetings, lasting one or two hours, are the means by which family goals can be decided, reviewed, and revised. Four major categories of family goals to improve eating and activity practices are recommended. For each category, *recommended* healthy goals are listed, based on research and professional advice.

At the initial family meeting, have family members decide on one goal from each of the four goal categories.

- Strive to increase or decrease your present practices in small steps until they match the recommended goals.

- A recommended time frame is to set healthy goals on a three-month basis.
- After three months, decide whether the healthy goals were met, whether one or more needs to be continued, or whether one or more new goals can be set.
- If a goal was not met, have members identify the problems that prevented it from being achieved and brainstorm ways to overcome the problems.
- Initial goals need to be achieved before additional ones are attempted.
- Be sure to mark on your calendar a date for a family meeting at the end of this three-month period.
- Over time, work hard on all the healthy goals that need improving.

The four goal categories with their recommended goals are described here.

Category One: Improving the Nutritional Quality of Dietary Intakes

- Consume two or three servings (depending upon age) of milk, other dairy products, or other calcium-rich sources daily.
- Consume at least five servings of fruits and vegetables daily, including a vitamin C-rich fruit or vegetable daily and a vitamin A-rich fruit or vegetable at least three times weekly.
- Consume at least three servings of whole-grain products daily.

Category Two: Promoting Healthy Eating Practices

- Eat a meal with the family, a "family meal," at least five days weekly.
- Eat three regular meals and one to three snacks consisting mainly of nutritious foods and beverages daily.
- Eat appropriate portion sizes of foods and beverages at meals and snacks daily, at and away from home, unless feelings of hunger indicate more or less.

- Eat and drink at a slow and steady pace so that major meals last daily, at or away from home, twenty to thirty minutes.
- Reduce intake of high-calorie, sweetened beverages (including soft drinks) to no more than one cup or can for adults daily; one cup or can for teens three or four days weekly; one cup or one can for school-age children two or three days weekly; and a half cup or can for preschool-age children two or three days weekly.
- Reduce the intake of high-calorie foods (high in fat, sweetened-type foods, and salty snack products, including sweets, desserts, and pastries) to one serving at one meal or snack no more than three or four days weekly for adults, teens, and school-age children; half of a serving two or three days weekly for preschool-age children; and a quarter serving one or two days weekly for infants and toddlers.
- Reduce eating meals and snacks in rooms other than the kitchen and dining area and while doing other activities to two or three days weekly.
- Eat only one meal or snack at a restaurant or fast-food establishment no more than two days weekly.
- Avoid overeating because of depression, stress, or other strong emotions at any time.

Category Three: Encouraging Physical Activity

- Do sixty minutes of a moderate-intensity **(**or vigorous**)** physical activity daily.
- Do stretching and strengthening activities, each for twenty minutes daily, on two or three days weekly.
- Reduce time spent watching television and on the computer for entertainment to no more than two hours daily.
- Reduce inactive times (such as reading or talking on the telephone) to no more than a half hour daily
- Plan a family-centered activity at least once monthly or as often as possible.

Category Four: Increasing Nutrition Knowledge

- Plan a nutrition education activity (at least one hour) monthly, or
- Plan a nutrition education activity (at least two hours) monthly.

Monitoring Healthy Goals

The purpose of monitoring (or tracking) is to determine whether healthy goals are met and maintained. For such monitoring, refer to the "Meeting Healthy Goals" on the following page.

- Throughout the three-month period, have family members keep track of whether or not they have met the healthy goals.
- Regarding nutrition education activities, determine whether this healthy goal has been met for the month.
- You may wish to create and reproduce "Meeting Healthy Goals" by hand or by a computer method of choice.
- Keep the "Meeting Healthy Goals" in order to compare them with future ones.

Meeting Healthy Goals

Remember to increase or decrease your present practices in small steps until they match the recommended goals. Write down the four family goals decided upon by family members. For example:

- Goal 1—add one serving of whole-grain products daily
- Goal 2—reduce high-calorie foods at one meal or snack once weekly
- Goal 3—every two weeks, increase moderate-intensity activity by fifteen minutes daily
- Goal 4—participate in a one-hour nutrition education activity monthly.

Circle (or place a gold star over) the days of the week in which the first three goals are met. For goal 4, circle (or place a gold star over) the week in which the nutrition education activity was conducted.

Goal 1:

_____

   Week 1: M T W TH F S Su
   Week 2: M T W TH F S Su
   Week 3: M T W TH F S Su
   Week 4: M T W TH F S Su

Goal 2:

_____

   Week 1: M T W TH F S Su
   Week 2: M T W TH F S Su
   Week 3: M T W TH F S Su
   Week 4: M T W TH F S Su

Goal 3:

_____

   Week 1: M T W TH F S Su
   Week 2: M T W TH F S Su
   Week 3: M T W TH F S Su
   Week 4: M T W TH F S Su

Goal 4:

_____

   Monthly: Week 1 Week 2 Week 3 Week 4

Choose My Plate: A Valuable Internet Evaluation Resource

Explore the "Choose My Plate" website (www.choosemyplate.gov). Based on my experience doing the following three activities at this website, the following steps are suggested:

- Click on Super Tracker & Other Tools.
- Then click on BMI calculator; look for children and teens and for adults. Enter the date of birth and the date of assessment (date calculating BMI), which provides a person's age for analysis. Then, enter height and weight. This will provide helpful tips for each weight status.
- Click on Food Tracker. The tracking of food and beverage intakes (and activity) have time limitations. Because of this, before starting, write down a typical day's dietary intake, including the foods and beverages eaten at each meal and snack and the amounts. If a food or beverage is purchased at a fast-food establishment, write down the name of the establishment before the food or beverage purchased. Calories for each food and beverage, total calories for the day, and a comparison with current dietary recommendations will be given.

Then, click on Physical Activity Tracker. Beforehand, write down a typical week of activities, including all activities, the type, and the number of minutes spent for each. A comparison with current physical activity recommendations will be presented.

These three educational tasks have been designed by nutrition professionals. They are user-friendly. Family members should complete these tasks at the beginning and every three months. Have each member save the findings of the three activities in order to compare results with subsequent six-month evaluations.

Monitoring Weights

Preventing obesity is a lifelong battle. Parents and children need to continue efforts to maintain the changes that have brought about the desired weight status. By monitoring weight, you can determine whether the family goals selected are insufficient, right on target, or too drastic in terms of weight control. This information can place you in a better position to guide family members to revise family goals at the next family meeting.

Weight checks should be done for children and teens every two weeks or on a monthly basis. Daily or weekly weight checks could place too much focus on weight or initiate a preoccupation with weighing. Keep a record of weights (date and weight).

Explain to your overweight or obese child or teen that it is important for everyone to do weight checks in order to be and stay healthy. This is to help your child or teen understand that you do not disapprove of him or her because of his or her weight. If a child's or teen's weight stays the same or increases when weight loss is desired, it is important to give a hug and say that you love him or her. Then, emphasize that the best hope for the family is to eat healthy and keep active, so just try harder next time. Parents may wish to help younger children with the recording of information. Older children and teens may prefer to keep these records themselves. Making healthy goals for the family removes the focus and pressure from a child or teen with a weight problem.

Recommended Nutrition-Related Activities

Most television commercials (especially those on Saturday mornings) and Internet advertisements promote unhealthy foods and beverages. The early establishment of healthy eating and activity behaviors practiced throughout the years can help children and teens resist the media and peer pressure to eat unwisely. For older children and teens, it is important to emphasize that adopting healthy eating and activity practices will not only be beneficial to his or her health but also that he or she will be a powerful role model for younger siblings.

Rather than the old saying "If you can't beat them, join them," think of the saying "If you can't beat them, have them join you." Invite your child's or teen's closest friends, cousins, or classmates to your monthly nutrition-related activities.

Suggestions for monthly nutrition-related activities are listed as follows:

❑ Review the recommended number of servings and serving sizes in the USDA Food Guide recommendations (chapter 1).

☐ Discuss healthy ways to prepare nourishing foods.

☐ Compare the contents of television commercials and Internet advertisements that they have seen during the month in terms of the nutritional value of the products and what is used to attract attention. (Beforehand, ask your children and teens to jot down notes about the commercial and advertisements.)

☐ Search for new recipes from a variety of cookbooks or the Internet and compare them in terms of nutritional value.

☐ Gather commercial products from cabinets, refrigerator, and freezer and compare them in terms of nutritional quality, according to the nutrition label.

☐ Discuss the present recommendations for increasing physical activity and decreasing sedentary pursuits. (Recommendations can be found in chapter 2.)

☐ Participate in nutrition-related websites and nutrition education-related printed information, videos, and games recommended by professional nutrition education resources. Some are given in the following points.

Ask for suggestions from family members, and create your own nutrition-related activities.

Nutrition Education Websites

A number of excellent websites provide helpful information.

Visit www.nationalheartlungandbloodinstitute.org/wecango slow andwhoafoods. Use the search option to find the "Go, Slow, and Whoa Foods." This division of foods and beverages was developed by the Coordinated Approach to Child Health program (www.catchinfo. org/about/wecangoslowandwhoafoods). Go foods and beverages are the most nourishing, such as fat-free and low-fat milk and whole-grain bread. Slow foods and beverages are less nourishing, such as 2 percent milk and white bread. Whoa foods and beverages are least nourishing, such as whole milk and pastries.

The following are also interesting websites:

- www.nationaldairycouncil.org (information on dairy products to meet calcium requirements)
- www.fiveaday.org (information about fruits and vegetables)
- www.bellinstitute.com/wholegrainkids—The "Go with the Whole Grain for Kids" information features two entertaining "Whole Grain Heroes" to help students learn about the benefits of whole grains. This fun and engaging curriculum is available in two versions: one for children in grades K–2 and one that is a more in-depth version for older children.
- www.foodchamps.org and www.fruitsandveggiesmore matters.org. These two highly praised web sources were developed by the Produce for Better Health Foundation (www.pbhcatalog.org).
- The Food Champs website offers a variety of interactive games, downloadable coloring sheets, activities, and kid-friendly recipes, while teaching kids about the importance of fruits and vegetables in meals and snacks.
- The Fruits and Veggies More Matters website (www.fruitsandveggiesmorematters.org) provides an extensive recipe database, a "What's in Season?" section, and tips on getting kids to eat more fruits and vegetables.

Children learning from a nutrition education web resource

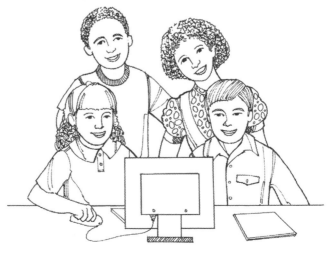

Chapter 10

Promoting Family Responsibility and Health

It is important that children and teens, girls and boys alike, participate in meal-related activities. These meal-related skills learned as children and teens can be very helpful when they become independent adults and/or when they become parents themselves. Being at ease in the kitchen and at the grocery store can reduce stress when they are called upon to use the meal-related skills as adults.

Family Responsibilities Related to the Planning and Preparing of Healthy Meals and Snacks

As emphasized previously, children and teens need to participate in activities related to the planning and preparing of healthy meals and snacks. Parents should ask each child or teen to participate in at least three different family responsibilities weekly; for example, helping to plan menus, finding coupons, and helping to prepare dinner.

Nine recommended family responsibilities are as follows:

1. Survey stores for nutritious products by comparing nutrition labels, such as lower-fat varieties or products with higher fiber content.
2. Plan healthy meals and snacks.
3. Create grocery lists from these menu plans.
4. Acquire coupons for healthy foods and beverages from newspapers or the Internet.
5. Participate in one or two shopping trips weekly.

6. Prepare healthy meals and snacks.
7. Help to clean up after meals and snacks.
8. Fix healthy bag lunches for lunch for work or school.
9. Help to prepare healthy recipes.

Keep in mind that you may wish to survey stores every six months to determine whether new, healthier products have become available. When surveying local stores for healthy foods and beverages and planning regular, balanced meals and snacks, alert other family members to the dates and times you plan these tasks so that as many members as possible can participate.

When doing your menu planning, remember to designate the meals that are to be "family meals." Designate the meals and snacks to be ordered from or eaten at restaurants or fast-food establishments, and coordinate your menus with weekly school lunch selections (or day care meals and snacks, if children participate).

Prepare healthy bag lunches for work and lunch the night before to help prevent adding to the morning rush.

For each responsibility, there is a recommended time and points assigned to acquire rewards. Such rewards not only encourage family members to do the activities but also helps them recognize the achievements once the activities have been successfully completed.

Monitoring Family Responsibilities

To help family members keep track of their participation in family responsibilities on a monthly basis, children and teens could use a log format in a spiral notebook (or on the computer), where they can record the following:

- date
- the type of activity
- the time spent on that activity
- points earned (to be described shortly)

This will help determine whether the responsibility has been met, and a reward can be given.

Rewarding Children and Teens

Every once in a while, remember to praise your child or teen so that he or she will continue participating in the meal-related activities. Rewards should be those that parents are willing and able to give, such as special privileges (for example, staying up an hour later) or parents participating in a favorite activity with the child or teen. Give rewards when responsibilities are met and withhold them when they are not. Meeting the responsibility means that the child or teen does the three specific family responsibilities each week. Rewards should not involve giving high-calorie foods and beverages.

Recommended Family Responsibilities

An average recommended time is suggested for each of the three activities per week. Each activity has been assigned points, which, once the activity has been completed, can be used to acquire a reward. At this time, stop and review the activities given below with their assigned point values.

- Help survey favorite stores (only two per month). Fifteen points for each store.
- Help develop a weekly menu plan (at least one hour) or menu plans for every two weeks (at least two hours). Ten points for each week's plan.
- Help create a grocery list for each week's menu plan (fifteen to twenty minutes for each week's list). Five points for each list.
- Help obtain coupons for healthy foods and beverages from newspapers or the Internet (ten to thirty minutes). Five points for each source.
- Help make one or two major shopping visits to the grocery stores (at least one hour each). Ten points for each visit.
- Help prepare a nourishing breakfast (ten to fifteen minutes), lunch (twenty to thirty minutes), dinner (twenty to thirty minutes), or a snack (ten to fifteen minutes). Do a variety. Ten points for each meal or snack.

- Help clean up after breakfast (ten minutes), lunch (fifteen minutes), dinner (twenty minutes), and snack (ten minutes). Do a variety. Five points for each cleanup.
- Prepare a healthy bagged lunch for work or school (ten to fifteen minutes). Five points for each lunch.
- Help prepare healthy recipes (thirty or sixty minutes) (one recipe per week). Fifteen points for each recipe.

After each four weeks, if you have acquired a minimum of one hundred points, select from one of the given rewards, modify rewards, or create new rewards. Extra points can be applied to the second four weeks. The following rewards are suggested:

1. Use sixty minutes to participate each week in a favorite activity, shared by the child and a parent.
2. Apply sixty minutes toward a special privilege each week.

If the above reward/point approach is not workable for your family at this time, an alternative is to have three or more family responsibilities done by children and teens serve as the basis or part of a weekly allowance. For this purpose, you may wish to use the log method to record the family responsibilities selected, time spent on that activity, and the dates they were done.

Chapter 11

Summary of Recommendations to Promote Healthy Eating and Activity Practices

The best way to teach your family healthy eating and activity practices is by adopting them yourself. It would be very difficult for you to successfully promote the following recommendations if you do not practice and reinforce them by being a positive role model. The recommendations can correct existing weight problems, but to prevent weight problems, it would be best to establish healthy eating and activity practices during the very early years of life. Keep in mind the wise words of Benjamin Franklin: "An ounce of prevention is worth a pound of cure." The recommendations have been designed to strike a balance between being too controlling and too flexible in terms of children's feeding practices.

❐ Prepare balanced meals and snacks that include foods and beverages from all the USDA's recommended food groups. Promote fruits and vegetables and whole-grain products, the two food groups that are most often lower than the recommended levels in the diets of children and teens.

❐ Offer a variety of foods and beverages at meals and snacks over time to broaden children's acceptance of nourishing foods and beverages, but also routinely offer the high-calorie foods and sweetened beverages that are children's favorites. Explain to children and teens that all foods and beverages are welcome but that how often they can be eaten differs. To help with this, read and discuss the "Go, Slow, and Whoa Foods." In addition, share with them the recommendations regarding high-calorie foods and beverages. Do not use high-calorie foods and beverages to reward, to punish by withdrawing them, or to comfort.

☐ Offer foods and beverages in moderation at meals and snacks—that is, in appropriate portion sizes—and allow children to eat more or less, depending upon their internal signals of hunger and being full. Smaller dishware and appropriate-sized glassware can present appropriate sizes in a realistic perspective.

☐ Encourage children to eat in response to their internal feelings of hunger and being full by using such techniques as "Your Energy Gauge." Praise your children and teens when they act upon such internal feelings.

☐ Slow down the pace of eating, if necessary, by encouraging smaller bites and chewing each bite well. Have children and teens pause a minute or so, once or more, during the meal or snack. Work hard to have major meals last between twenty and thirty minutes.

☐ Strongly encourage participation in family meals. At the same time, reduce the number of meals and snacks that are eaten outside of the home.

☐ Have children and teens participate in a wide variety of physical activities that are safe, age appropriate, and of interest. Strongly encourage at least sixty minutes daily of a moderate-intensity activity and at least twenty minutes daily each for strengthening and stretching activities on two or three days weekly. At the same time, reduce sedentary activities, such as watching TV or using the computer for entertainment purposes, to no more than two hours daily, and time spent on other inactive pursuits, including talking or texting on the phone, to no more than a half hour daily. Plan family-based activities.

The last important recommendation is to promote healthy eating and activity practices in terms of healthy goals for the family. Explain to your children and teens that improvements in their eating and activity practices are the goals to becoming a healthier family.

Index

chronic diseases, 75, 81
computer time, importance of
limiting of, 34–35
Cooperative Extension Service, 37
Coordinated Approach to Child
Health program, 104
cow's milk, 16
cup, introducing use of, 13

D

dairy products. *See also* milk group
recommended intake of for
preschoolers, 20–21*t*
recommended intake of for
school-age children and
teens, 24
recommended intake of for
toddlers, 17*t*
diabetes, type 2, 75, 79
Dietary Guidelines for Americans
(2015), 59
dietary plans, for children and
teens, 91–95

E

eating
pace of, 3, 48, 112
reducing eating in rooms other
than kitchen and dining
room while doing other
activities, 52
eating disorders, 76, 96, 97
eating practices
of children as mirroring those
of parents, xvi
recommended frequency of,
44–45
emotional overeating, reduction of,
54–55
emotional problems, associated
with weight difficulties, 75

energy equation, 43, 57
energy gauge, 46–47, 55, 112
engorgement (when breast-
feeding), 2
environmental influences, and
weight problems, 80
excess weight
cause of, 43
steps to prevent/correct excess
weight in preschool and
school-age children and
teens, 82–90

F

fad diets, cautions with, 80
family meals, importance of, 32–33
family responsibilities
monitoring of, 108
promotion of, 107–110
recommendations for, 109–110
related to planning/
preparation of healthy
meals and snacks,
107–108
fast-food establishments/
restaurants, decreasing
meals and snacks taken in,
52–54
fats and oils
recommended intake of for
preschoolers, 20–21*t*
recommended intake of for
school-age children and
teens, 27
recommended intake of for
toddlers, 17*t*
five Hs, xvi
fiveaday.org (website), 106
folate, 30
folic acid, 30
Food Champs (website), 106

high-calorie foods
in diets of infants and toddlers, 18
in diets of preschoolers, 22
in diets of school-age children and teens, 28–29
reducing intake of, 48–50
hunger
becoming tuned in to internal feelings of, 45–47
common actions of infants who are hungry, 8
hypertension, 79

I

infant feeding practices
breast-feeding, 1–2, 3, 7, 12, 13, 14, 15, 37
formula-feeding, 1, 2, 3, 7, 8, 11, 12, 13, 14, 15, 37, 70
during growth spurts, 2
healthy practices, 3–4
infant foods, homemade, 5
infant foods, introduction of, 3–4, 11, 12–14
minimizing risk of choking, 4, 9, 11
pace of eating, 2–3
practices to avoid, 3
sample daily plan, 11–15
infants. *See also* infant feeding practices
actions of infants who express hunger and being full, 7–8
evaluation of growth in, 65–66
healthy food and beverage intakes for, 8–9
high-calorie foods in diets of, 18
promotion of healthy weight in, 63–74
rapid growth in, 64
recommended dietary intakes for, 6–18
reducing risk of overfeeding of, 6
steps to prevent/correct excess weight in, 67–70
iron, importance of, 30

J

Jones, Elizabeth, xvii, 3, 5, 13, 63

L

laboratory testing, 79

M

mastitis, 2
McCormick, Kimberly, 37
meals
for children, 35–37
decreasing meals taken in fast-food establishments/restaurants, 52–54
family responsibilities related to planning/preparation of, 107–108
importance of sharing of, 32–33
participating in family responsibilities related to, 39–40
recommendations for eating regular meals, 45
for teens, 37–38
measurements, table of equal measurements, 7t
meat and meat alternatives
healthy intakes of for infants, 10–11
recommended intake of for preschoolers, 20–21t

recommended intake of for
school-age children and
teens, 24–25
recommended intake of for
toddlers, 17t
medical information, importance of
keeping records of, 79
milk group, healthy intakes of for
infants, 8
mineral supplements, cautions
with, 29
moderate-intensity activities, 60
moderation, principle, 44

N

National Dairy Council, 106
nursing, 1. *See also* breast-feeding
nutrition education websites,
105–106
nutrition labels, teaching children
and teens about, 40–42
nutrition-related activities, 104–105

O

Obama, Michelle, 6
obese
percent of US children and
teens that are, 6
use of term, xv
overweight
steps to prevent/correct excess
weight in infants and
toddlers, 67–68
use of term, xv
oxidants, 23

P

pace of eating, 3, 48, 112
parenting/parents
and correcting unhealthy
feeding practices, 43–56

and promoting healthy eating
practices, 31–42
and promoting healthy
physical activity
practices, 57–62
role of in establishing healthy
practices in children, xvi
unhealthy parental feeding
practices, 31–32
physical activities, benefits of, 60
physical fitness
becoming physically fit as a
family, 58–59
guidelines for encouragement
of, 59–60
physical activity plan for your
family, 60–62
places for eating, reducing eating
in rooms other than kitchen
and dining room while doing
other activities, 52
portion sizes
having children take own as
they become older, 31
importance of paying attention
to, 6, 7, 22–23, 49, 99, 112
large portion sizes as
unhealthy eating
practice, xvi, 94
reduction of, 47–48
positive examples, by parents,
caregivers, and older
siblings, 44
praise, importance of, 56, 109
pregnancy, recommendations
for weight changes during,
63–64
preschool children
healthy food and beverage
intakes for, 19–21
high-calorie foods in diets of, 22

Printed in the United States
By Bookmasters